Affordable Excellence:
The Singapore Healthcare Story

Affordable Excellence:
The Singapore Healthcare Story

How to Create and Manage Sustainable Healthcare Systems

William A. Haseltine

Brookings Institution Press
Washington, D.C.

ABOUT BROOKINGS

The Brookings Institution is a private nonprofit organization devoted to research, education, and publication on important issues of domestic and foreign policy. Its principal purpose is to bring the highest quality independent research and analysis to bear on current and emerging policy problems. Interpretations or conclusions in Brookings publications should be understood to be solely those of the authors.

Affordable Excellence: The Singapore Healthcare Story may be ordered from:
Brookings Institution Press
1775 Massachusetts Avenue, N.W.
Washington, D.C. 20036
Telephone: 1-800/537-5487 or 410/516-6956
E-mail: hfscustserv@press.jhu.edu; www.brookings.edu/press

This edition is not for sale in Asia, Australia, or New Zealand.

Simultaneously published by Ridge Books, an imprint of NUS Press, National University of Singapore, AS3-01-02, 3 Arts Link, Singapore 117569

Library of Congress Cataloging-in-Publication data is available
ISBN: 978-0-8157-2416-2 (pbk. : alk. paper)

9 8 7 6 5 4 3 2 1

Printed on acid-free paper

Composition by Forum
Kuala Lumpur, Malaysia

Printed by Versa Press
East Peoria, Illinois

Contents

List of Illustrations

Tables

Chapter 3

Chapter 7

Charts

Chapter 2

Chapter 3

The author has resolved all copyright issues related to material in this publication.

Acknowledgments

This book was inspired by a speech given in 2010 by then Minister for Health of Singapore, Khaw Boon Wan, to an international group of health specialists. I had the good fortune to attend the meeting of NIHA (the Initiative to Improve Health in Asia), a Pan-Asian Policy Program sponsored by the National University of Singapore and the Global Asia Institute. The Minister's speech outlined the history and more importantly, the thinking, behind the creation of the Singapore healthcare system. The system he described is both effective and unique. I asked if a book existed describing the Singapore approach to healthcare and was surprised to learn that none did. A few weeks later, I had a follow-up conversation over dinner with the NUS President, Tan Chorh Chuan, Director of the Global Asia Institute, Seetharam Kallidaikurichi Easwaran, and Paul Kratoska, then Director of NUS Press who encouraged me to write this volume. Seetharam Kallidaikurichi kindly provided support for a researcher for a year and the book was on its way. I mentioned that I was writing a volume on the Singapore healthcare system that might provide lessons in the creation of sustainable healthcare system to others in both developing and developed countries to Strobe Talbott of the Brookings Institution, and he and his colleagues kindly offered to jointly publish the book with NUS Press. I am grateful to Robert Faherty, Director of the Brookings Press for his encouragement. I thank Peter Schoppert, now Director of NUS Press, for his enthusiasm and assistance.

I owe special thanks to Claudia Olsson, Managing Director of ACCESS Health International, Singapore for her valuable assistance throughout. She organized interviews for me, conducted others herself, did much of the research for the final chapter of the book and worked closely with our researcher, Eti Bhaskar. Eti was tireless in preparing background material for each chapter and tracking down the necessary information. I owe her a deep debt of gratitude.

Both the Ministry of Health and the Singapore Economic Development Board were very helpful. The current Minister Gan Kim Yong graciously allowed us to interview him and his colleagues at the Ministry. Both helped to arrange the numerous interviews with key players in the healthcare system, both public and private, as well as past and present. Special thanks go to Lee Chien Earn, former Head of the Department of Public Health and Deputy Chief Medical Officer of the Ministry of Health and Lim Eng Kok, Deputy Director (Service Management) of the Ministry of Health, for their continued assistance and help in identifying people and documents important for this story. Representatives from the Ministry of Health graciously responded to my long series of written questions. I have cited this material and reproduced some of these answers in the Appendix of this volume.

I list here many of the people who were kind enough to grant us interviews, without which we would not have been able to assemble the remarkable story of the Singapore healthcare system past and present. They were to a person helpful in all ways and patient in answering our questions.

These include: Tan See Leng, Group CEO and Managing Director of Parkway Pantai Limited; Tan Ser Kiat, Chairman of SingHealth Foundation; Chee Yam Cheng, Group CEO of National Healthcare Group; Yong Ying-I, Previous Permanent Secretary for Health; Yee Ping Yi, CEO of the CPF Board; Sarah Muttitt, former CIO, Information Systems Division, MOH Holdings; K. Ranga Rama Krishnan, Dean, Duke-NUS Graduate Medical School; Edward Holmes, A*STAR Executive Deputy Chairman, Biomedical Research Council; Phua Kai Hong, Associate Professor of Health Policy and Management, Lee Kuan Yew School of Public Policy; Chia Kee Seng, Dean, NUS Saw Swee Hock School of Public Health; Jason Cheah, CEO, Agency for Integrated Care; Wong Loong Mun, Chief Care Integration Officer, Agency for Integrated Care (AIC); C. Frank Starmer, Associate Dean for Learning Technologies, Duke-NUS Graduate Medical School; Lim Chuan Poh, A*STAR Chairman; John Lim, CEO, Health Sciences Authority; Chua Song Khim, Group CEO of China Healthcare Ltd; Anthony Tan, former Director of the Healthcare Finance and Corporate Services of the Ministry of Health; Ang Hak Seng, CEO of the Health Promotion Board; John Wong, former Dean of the NUS Yong Loo Lin School of Medicine; Benjamin Ong, Chief Executive of the National University Health System; Elizabeth Koh, former Group Director (People Matters) and Senior Director (Healthcare Leadership

Development), Ministry of Health; Elizabeth Quah, Group Director (Planning), Ministry of Health; Peter Lee, former Deputy Director of the Learning Systems Standards & Quality Improvement Division, and the Organizational Excellence Corporate Human Resource Division, Ministry of Health; David Matchar, Professor and Director, Program in Health Services and Systems Research, Duke-NUS Graduate Medical School; Tan Yong Seng, Chairman, People's Association Active Ageing Council; Mary Ann Tsao, President, Tsao Foundation; Susana Concordo Harding, Director, International Longevity Centre Singapore, Tsao Foundation; Phua Puay Li, Director, Manpower Planning & Strategy Division, Ministry of Health; Martyn R. Partridge, Senior Vice Dean, Lee Kong Chian School of Medicine; Lim Siong Guan, Group President, Government of Singapore Investment Corporation; Denise Lee, Manager (Clinical Benchmarking), Performance and Technology Assessment Division (PTA), Ministry of Health; Kishore Mahbubani, Dean and Professor in the Practice of Public Policy of the Lee Kuan Yew School of Public Policy at NUS.

Others who provided support and assistance thoughout the research and writing include: Lee Suet-Fern, Senior Director, Stamford Law Corporation; Min-Tze Lean, Director, Stamford Law Corporation; Bernard Yeung, Dean at NUS Business School; Sofi Bergkvist, Managing Director, ACCESS Health International; and Priya Anant, CFO, ACCESS Health International.

I am grateful to support from ACCESS Health International, a not-for-profit operating foundation dedicated to promoting access to high-quality and affordable health worldwide, of which I am Chairman and President. The proceeds from this book will be going in their entirety to supporting its work.

My thanks also go to my very good friend Ambassador Chan Heng Chee. Over the many years we have known each other, she has worked tirelessly on behalf of her country. Starting many years ago, she introduced me to key decision-makers in Singapore from all walks of life. She, more than any other person, is the inspiration for this volume. It is my hope that others will find lessons in the Singapore healthcare story and experience to apply in their own countries to improve the lives and health of their citizens.

Finally, I thank Dave Conti for his valuable editorial assistance and constant input throughout the writing of this book.

William A. Haseltine
Washington, DC, April 2013

Introduction

Why this book? *Affordable Excellence* tells the story of the Singapore healthcare system, how it works, how it is financed, its history, and where it is going.

Today Singapore ranks sixth in the world in healthcare outcomes well ahead of many developed countries, including the United States. The results are all the more significant as Singapore spends less on healthcare than any other high-income country, both as measured by fraction of the Gross Domestic Product spent on health and by costs per person. Singapore achieves these results at less than one-fourth the cost of healthcare in the United States and about half that of Western European countries. Government leaders, presidents and prime ministers, finance ministers and ministers of health, policymakers in congress and parliament, public health officials responsible for healthcare systems planning, finance and operations, as well as those working on healthcare issues in universities and think-tanks should know how this system works to achieve affordable excellence.

The lessons from Singapore should be of interest to those currently planning the future of healthcare in emerging economies, for Singapore was not always rich. In just 50 years, Singapore transformed itself from a low-income country to one that has one of the highest per capita incomes in the world, from a country with poor health outcomes to one of the best in the world. What was the philosophy and what were the key decisions that drove this transformation? Leaders and policy planners may well ask—will this work in my country?

One point that emerges clearly: decisions made early on affect the course of later history. Once begun, it is very difficult to revise health finance and delivery systems, as such decisions profoundly affect the lives of individuals and economies. To finance healthcare, should countries adopt a mixture of private and public insurance as does the United States, the state approach to healthcare finance and operations as in the United Kingdom, or the public–private partnerships of Germany and Japan? Or should an entirely different approach be taken, that of Singapore, where emphasis is placed on individual responsibility supported by an enabling state? *Affordable Excellence* describes the Singaporean approach as an alternative well worth considering.

Singapore also offers useful lessons for wealthy countries with long-established healthcare systems. The world's most developed countries are facing a crisis of confidence in their healthcare systems. Costs are rising at an alarming and seemly uncontrollable rate. In the United States, healthcare accounts for almost 18 percent of the GDP and is rising. Most developed economies are facing twin demographic problems: the population of the elderly is rising rapidly and the population of the young, who must support them, is shrinking. The cost of caring for the elderly far exceeds that for the young. Yet as earning power declines with age, it is not compensated for by increased earning capacity among the young.

The Singapore system offers a guide to controlling costs and paying for health in the present. It may also provide a blueprint for the future. Singapore is relatively unique amongst governments in its ability to plan for the future. In the past, the government has planned and successfully executed, over a 30-year period, strategies requiring the integration of the activities of most government ministries. That is how the current healthcare system was designed and built. Today, the emphasis is on planning for the coming demographic crises using the same cross-ministry approach that has worked so well in the past. How can the current system be adapted to provide excellent care for the elderly at a cost the country can afford? This is the central issue for all developed economies. Those planning for the future might well look to Singapore for ideas on how to prepare for the challenges ahead.

I was surprised to learn that no book describing the Singapore healthcare system has been written. To be sure, aspects of the system are described in many monographs and books that treat more general topics. *Affordable Excellence* provides a source for those wishing a more comprehensive knowledge of how the system was built, financed and operates. In writing this volume, I have often been told that Singapore is unique and lessons learned are not applicable elsewhere. Some say Singapore is small and solutions to problems there will not work elsewhere. Others believe only a government with a long tenure in power (Singapore's ruling People's Action Party has been in power since independence in 1965) can achieve comparable results. Some even go so far as to describe Singapore as a dictatorship—an inaccurate characterization in my view—and that such a healthcare system can only be imposed by a controlling government. My answer to these challenges is that I am a scientist trained to look at what works. We call working examples "proof of principle." The Singapore experiment does work, proving that healthcare systems can be designed that provide high-quality healthcare to all citizens in a highly-developed economy at a cost the economy can afford, and that costs can be controlled while delivering excellent service. True, the continuity and long-term perspective that come from political stability may make it easier for a government to develop a strong healthcare system (see next chapter); nonetheless, Singapore has much to teach health systems no matter what their political context.

CHAPTER 1

The Singapore Healthcare System: An Overview

Singapore has achieved extraordinary results both in the high quality of its healthcare system and in controlling the cost of care. In per capita terms and as a percentage of Gross Domestic Product (GDP), its healthcare expenditures are the lowest of all the high-income countries in the world.

How did this happen? How has Singapore been able to achieve these kinds of results?

The answers are bigger than just the process of putting a healthcare system together. There are larger factors that have to do with the spirit and philosophy of Singapore itself, the way it is governed, how the government approaches domestic issues, and how it deals with the world.

In my study of Singapore, I have found three compelling qualities woven into the fabric of the country that have enabled it to achieve outstanding successes in so many areas, healthcare included. They are long-term political unity, the ability to recognize and establish national priorities, and the consistent desire for collective well-being and social harmony of the country.

Political Unity and Constancy of Purpose

From the time the British withdrew from Singapore and left its former colony to fend for itself, Singapore has been able to develop and grow as an integrated whole. The People's Action Party (PAP) has been in power since independence, resulting in sustained political stability. Along with stability has come a unity and constancy of purpose and action throughout government. Contrast this condition with other countries where government regularly changes hands and different parties espousing different agendas go in and out of power. A clear and uninterrupted approach to solving a nation's problems is very difficult to achieve in such situations. The government has been steady in its broad general vision of what care should be and what role it should play in the lives of Singaporeans. That continuity of philosophy and approach, I believe, has made possible the ability to plan and execute over a long period of time.

I have also observed an unusual degree of unity among the country's various ministries—an acknowledged spirit of cooperation among governmental departments that makes possible the formulation of policies that reaches across ministries. A member of the team that assembled the 1983 health plan discussed in this chapter and Health Minister from 2004 to 2011, Mr. Khaw Boon Wan, has noted that each month, Permanent Secretaries of each ministry meet to focus on issues that require participation by more than one ministry.[1] It is simply assumed that ministers will work as a team on issues that need interdepartmental cooperation.

I find it relevant that the government realized early on that improvement in health conditions and care had to be approached as an integral and inseparable part of the overall development planning for the country. As a heavily urbanized city-state with a population of two million at independence, caring for the health of the people meant more than just building hospitals and clinics. Health would be affected by almost every aspect of life in an urban setting: housing, water supply, food supply, air quality, waste disposal, road traffic, parks, tree planting, and more. Ensuring the health of the people of Singapore had to be built into every aspect of urban planning, requiring a comprehensive approach and the cooperation of numerous ministries over all the various sectors of government. The culture of cooperation made it all possible.

Some have suggested that Singapore is a thinly-disguised dictatorship, and that political stability is attained at the cost of democratic freedom. That is simply not the case. Although one party, the PAP, has been in power since independence, it is elected and does not hold power through force, and could not have maintained its rule without being highly responsive to the concerns of the electorate.

The government is responsive to the concerns of the electorate. In the 2011 elections, healthcare was one of the issues raised. There were concerns that the government was not doing enough for the elderly and that families were experiencing severe financial strain and even bankruptcy as they tried to pay for older family members' care. Opposition parties organized themselves around issues of healthcare affordability and eldercare costs.

Early the following year, the government responded with a new program of increased spending—doubling the Ministry of Health's budget over the next five years—to address citizens' concerns. It announced increased subsidies for long-term care, even for patients being cared for in the home, and expanded eligibilities for subsidies, giving middle-income families some financial relief. Subsidies were increased for nursing homes (including eligible patients in private nursing homes), day care, rehabilitation care, and home-based care. These actions by the government seem to me to be a direct response to the issues raised in the elections.

Establishing Priorities

The health of the populace was not a top priority for the government at the start of independence. As Lee Kuan Yew observed in his memoirs, he had three immediate concerns to deal with: international recognition for Singapore's independence; a strong defense program that would "defend this piece of real estate"; and finally the economy—"how to make a living for our people."[2] Yong Nyuk Lin, the Minister for Health at the time, stated the situation bluntly: "health would rank, at the most, fifth in order of priority" for public funds. National security, job creation, housing, and education were in the queue ahead of health, in that order.[3] With the exception of the basics of public health, healthcare planning and development would have to wait until the nation achieved a level of military and economic stability.

It seems to me that this ordering of priorities was apt for the time, as it was vitally important first to set up the defense of this small nation, and then to attract investors to set in motion economic growth, and tackle glaring issues of unemployment, housing, and education. After these critical problems had been dealt with, others, including healthcare, could be taken on. Exactly where health comes in the priorities of an emerging economy may vary. In countries where HIV/AIDS is highly prevalent, or if another epidemic or disease threatens a broad segment of the population, health may become the first or second national priority.

Wisely, the initial focus in Singapore was on public health: putting proper sanitation procedures in place, controlling infectious diseases, all successful efforts. Early initiatives were launched to provide clean water, develop a vaccination program, and guarantee access to basic medications, clean food, and more.

In time, the priorities set by the government proved to be effective. The security situation stabilized and the economy grew to the benefit of all. The creation of the healthcare system was aided immeasurably by the outstanding growth. One important indicator to consider: GDP grew from just under S$8.5 billion in 1964, to over S$50 billion in 1983 (the year the government issued its White Paper declaring its healthcare goals and which I will be discussing below), to almost S$300 billion in 2011.[4] Those economic gains were successfully translated into raising the health standards of the nation and building the care system that is the subject of this book.

Promoting a Sense of Collective Well-Being and Social Harmony

One of the most important tenets of Singaporean governance is that a strong society requires social harmony. If tensions between social groups and races are to be avoided, all groups should be included in the life of the country and should benefit, to some degree, from its successes. The government's actions on behalf of this belief have undergirded the building of modern Singapore. As part of the social fabric, the government built a system that promotes a sense of fairness and well-being through both economic opportunity and delivery of social services. I find these words of Lee key to understanding Singapore's approach:

> A competitive, winner-takes-all society, like colonial Hong Kong in the 1960s, would not be acceptable in Singapore ... To even out the extreme results of free-market competition, we had to redistribute the national income through subsidies on things that improved the earning power of citizens, such as education. Housing and public health were also obviously desirable. But finding the correct solutions for personal medical care, pensions, or retirement benefits was not easy.[5]

One important solution Lee and his ministers found was the Central Provident Fund (CPF). It was set up during British colonial rule as a compulsory savings program for workers to build a nest egg for retirement. Individuals put five percent of their wages into the fund and their employers matched it. The accumulated money could be withdrawn at age 55. Lee's government expanded the program, upping the contribution levels, and allowing funds to be used for home-buying (widespread home ownership was seen as vital for political and social stability).[6]

The CPF has become one of the key pillars supporting social stability. The government had a long-range vision to increase the use of the Fund over time and broaden it to allow individuals to save for and pay for education and healthcare as well as retirement and home-buying. Mandatory contribution rates have risen over the years and now stand at 16 percent of wage for employers and 20 percent for employees. After age 50, the rates decrease.

The Central Provident Fund's contribution to the viability of the healthcare system cannot be overstated: it helps control costs by instilling in patients a sense of responsibility about their spending—after all, it is their money to save or spend; and it helps make care available and affordable to all. Eventually, however, the government recognized that the health savings program would not be enough to support care, and other systems were put in place, including a medical insurance program and a social safety net.

Respect and Education for Women

The Central Provident Fund's contribution to the viability of the healthcare system cannot be overstated: it helps control costs by instilling in patients a sense of responsibility about their spending—after all, it is their money to save or spend; and it helps make care available and affordable to all. Eventually, however, the government recognized that the health savings program would not be enough to support care, and other systems were put in place, including a medical insurance program and a social safety net.

Specifically, women's health education was deemed essential to the future of the country. The Education Ministry took the lead in educating young women about important health topics. The then Health Minister Mr. Khaw Boon Wan credited that effort with creating a vitally important advance in healthcare: educated women were now able to look after their own health, their health during pregnancy, their babies, and their families.[7]

* * *

In the coming chapters, I will take you through these and other elements that have made healthcare in Singapore such an enviable achievement: the high quality of care, more on the critical role of the CPF, financing the system, controlling costs, infrastructure, investing in medical research, and the new challenges of long-term care and eldercare. But first, in the remainder of this chapter, I will walk you through the ideas and the history of social planning that created the foundation for today's healthcare system.

Singapore's transformation from a British colonial outpost to a First-World city-state is nothing short of remarkable. Since achieving independence in 1965 as a tiny, impoverished country with few assets and no natural resources, it has turned itself into a modern, prosperous, secure city-state.

Singapore's founding father, Lee Kuan Yew, knew that without Britain's military and financial support, this new country would succeed and endure only if it could turn itself into a "First World oasis in a Third World region."

Many institutions had to be erected before Singapore was able to reach that goal. How it was all accomplished makes for a fascinating study in nation-building. However, the scope of this book allows me to focus my discussion on the underlying Singaporean philosophy and actions that drove the development of the public healthcare system. While providing for the health needs of his people, Lee also wanted his country to avoid the pitfalls of Western systems—such as those in the United Kingdom and the United States—that were already showing signs of strain caused by high costs.

In the late 1940s, as a student at Cambridge, Lee witnessed the beginnings of the English welfare state:

> Looking back at those early years, I am amazed at my youthful innocence. I watched Britain at the beginning of its experiment with the welfare state; the Atlee government started to build a society that attempted to look after its citizens from cradle to grave. I was so impressed after the introduction of the National Health Service when I went to collect my pair of new glasses from my opticians in Cambridge to be told that no payment was due. All I had to do was to sign a form. What a civilised society, I thought to myself. The same thing happened at the dentist and the doctor.[8]

Over time, though, Lee realized that a system that took care of all of its citizens' needs would diminish the population's "desire to achieve and succeed." It was obvious to him that Singapore, upon independence, was a poor, struggling country that needed a motivated population working hard in the interests of their country and their future. He could not begin to contemplate a system like Britain's. If anything may be identified as the guiding philosophy behind Singapore's success, it is Lee's conviction that the people's desire to achieve and succeed must never be compromised by an overgenerous state. The government made certain that Singaporeans developed and retained a sense of responsibility for all aspects of their lives—including the care and maintenance of their own physical and emotional well-being.

Building the Foundation

Bringing Care to the People

I mentioned earlier that high-quality healthcare was not a high priority in the early days of independence. However the young government did take some significant steps to improve the health of Singaporeans. An early move was to bring primary care services closer to the people by developing a network of satellite outpatient dispensaries and maternal and child health clinics. They offered a one-stop center for immunization, health promotion, health screening, well-women programs, family planning services, nutritional advice, psychiatric counseling, dental care, pharmaceutical, x-ray, clinical laboratory, and even home-nursing and rehabilitative services for non-ambulatory patients.[9] The move took the pressure off Singapore's General Hospitals to provide such care.

Mr. Khaw Boon Wan characterized the movement to outpatient clinics as one of the low-hanging fruits in the transformation of the healthcare system, yielding a high return for a low investment, a necessary condition in the early days of the country.[10] These outpatient clinics have since been consolidated into modern polyclinics, small, well-equipped medical centers providing a range of diagnostic and treatment capabilities that do not require overnight stays, and catering to all age groups. Although acute illnesses still represent the majority of the problems being seen at polyclinics, the clinics are increasingly focused on chronic disease management. Services such as home-nursing and rehabilitative care for non-ambulatory patients have since been moved from polyclinics to Voluntary Welfare Organizations, community hospitals, and private nursing homes.

Introduction of User Fees at Public Clinics

Services at the outpatient clinics had been free-of-charge—modeled after the practice of the British healthcare system. But the government quickly changed that.

As Lee Kuan Yew recalled in his memoirs:

> The ideal of free medical services collided against the reality of human behaviour, certainly in Singapore. My first lesson came from government clinics and hospitals. When doctors prescribed free antibiotics, patients took their tablet or capsules for two days, did not feel better, and threw away the balance. They then consulted private doctors, paid for their antibiotics, completed the course, and recovered.

Lee's government imposed a fee of 50 cents for each attendance at the clinics, doubled during public holidays.[11] This bold move reminded Singaporeans that healthcare is not free, and that the nation would not be building a welfare system such as Britain's. People would be expected to a large degree to pay their own way.

Early Human Resources/Manpower Planning

Before 1960, there were fewer than 50 medical specialists in Singapore to serve Singapore's two million residents. To boost their numbers, the Committee for Postgraduate Medical Education was set up in 1970.[12] Initially, there were few specializations offered in Singapore. The government began sending its brightest doctors in the public sector to the best medical institutions around the world for training.

In the 1980s, the Healthcare Manpower Development Programme was launched giving specialists opportunities to work and train at world-renowned overseas institutes. HMDP at the outset was meant for specialist training, and subsequently subspecialty training was introduced in areas such as trauma, advanced cardiology techniques, gastro-pathology, breast reduction, and more.[13] This action nurtured a new generation of highly-skilled specialists and set the stage for developing Singapore's current world-class capability in highly-specialized, advanced medicine.

Over the years, Singapore has continued to forge strategic partnerships with healthcare organizations all around the world and continues to send doctors for training at world-class medical facilities. In 2009, 1,750 doctors practicing in Singapore were foreign-trained. Half of newly-recruited doctors are foreign-trained.[14]

Healthcare Infrastructure Improvements

Early on, the government began upgrading the infrastructure at public hospitals, all of which dated from before the Second World War. Gradually, one at a time, facilities were improved, investments were made in modern equipment, and sophisticated specialties were developed. Ambitious hospital construction and expansion programs have been undertaken since.[15] To encourage community participation and initiative in providing healthcare to the elderly, chronically sick, terminally ill, and mentally ill, the government began providing subsidies to certain private institutes and Voluntary Welfare Organizations and continues to do so today.

Housing

Although not a part of the healthcare system per se, the country's early housing initiative has contributed immeasurably to the health of Singaporeans. I would be remiss in not mentioning it here.

In the days before independence, according to the Housing and Development Board (HDB), many Singaporeans were living in "unhygienic slums and crowded squatter settlements."[16] At the time, only nine percent of Singaporeans lived in government flats. Set up in 1960, HDB began investing in good, clean affordable housing that greatly improved living conditions and health conditions. In less than three years, over 20,000 flats were built. By 1965, the number climbed to almost 55,000 flats, and within ten years, the housing problem was solved.[17] Today almost 85 percent of Singaporeans live in HDB flats. I believe that this effort on behalf of the people remains one of the most successful examples of public housing in the world.

For anyone interested in learning about living conditions before the improvements I have just discussed, I highly recommend a visit to the Chinatown Heritage Centre at 48 Pagoda Street. There visitors will find a fascinating recreation of housing from the 1950s, including reconstructed interiors.

The government did not stop at providing housing. Over the years, other investments were made in clean water, proper sanitation services, clean environment, good nutrition, and health education. All these actions played a crucial role in improving the health status of Singaporeans.[18]

Affordable Healthcare for All

In 1983, almost two decades after independence, the first comprehensive National Health Plan was introduced. The plan presented the government's broad health development strategies including keeping care affordable, meeting the demands of a growing population, and managing the rising expectations of an increasingly affluent society. It set national objectives for empowering Singaporeans to lead healthy, fit, and productive lives made possible through active disease prevention and promotion of a healthy lifestyle. The plan aimed to improve cost-efficiency in the system. Interestingly, it foresaw the growing demand for increased care for the rapidly ageing population.[19] The plan mentioned the need to restructure the healthcare delivery system to cope with the changing trends of diseases— mainly the shift from treating infectious disease to chronic disease.[20] The plan reflected the success of the early measures taken by the government to contain infectious diseases, provide clean water, and promote childhood vaccinations, allowing the focus of efforts to shift to chronic diseases. In time, Singapore began focusing on disease prevention through a healthy lifestyle—including exercise, eating healthy, managing stress, stopping smoking—along with screening for and optimal treatment of disease.[21] In this respect, Singapore was well in advance of other countries in the region that only started to shift their emphasis to chronic diseases around 2010 or so.

Restructuring

A sweeping reform started in the 1980s, when the government embarked upon the restructuring of its public hospitals, giving them greater autonomy to function more like private hospitals than public institutions under a central control. Speaking as an entrepreneur, I can imagine how liberating this move must have felt to hospital management. National University Hospital was incorporated in 1985, and Singapore General Hospital was incorporated in 1989. The majority of the hospitals were corporatized in the 1990s. The goal was to allow the public hospitals to compete against one another. The unsubsidized wards were meant to serve as a benchmark in terms of quality and price for the private sector. This action helped stabilize prices throughout the system.

The public hospitals were given a freer hand to implement management practices for improving effectiveness and efficiency, and much more freedom in their day-to-day decisions regarding staffing, compensation, deployment of resources, and some user fees. The reforms succeeded in providing consumers with more choices for their healthcare and also served to dampen rising costs. The public hospitals are still owned by the Ministry of Health through a holding company called the Health Corporation of Singapore set up in 1985. It later became MOH Holdings Private Limited. The government appoints the Board members, and the Chief Executive Officers and management of the hospitals are accountable to the Board, allowing the government to continue to exercise its authority in larger, strategic decision-making.[22]

Medisave

Perhaps most importantly, the Plan announced the creation of Medisave, Singapore's individual medical savings plan. Medisave is the expansion of the Central Provident Fund mentioned earlier in the chapter. Workers contribute a certain percentage (set by the government) to their individual accounts, as do their employers. The money can then be used to pay for health services as well as health insurance plans. I firmly believe that the program is one of the cornerstones of the current system. Medisave enables patients to pay their share of their healthcare bill. It has also had the effect of keeping national healthcare costs low by shifting a large portion of expenses to individuals and their employers. I discuss Medisave in depth in Chapter 3.

Blueprint for a Modern Healthcare System

By the early 1990s, it became clear that healthcare costs were growing at an alarming rate that would soon put an unacceptable strain on the nation's as well as family finances. It was also recognized that increasing life expectancy was creating another challenge: how to care for the growing elderly population in Singapore. A Ministerial Committee was set up to review the role the government could play in containing costs, controlling subsidies, and ensuring the continued quality of care. In 1993, the committee issued its report in a White Paper entitled "Affordable Health Care."[23]

The White Paper became, in effect, the blueprint for developing and refining a healthcare system that would serve the population well into the 21st century. In outlining the government's philosophy and approach to healthcare, it set forth five fundamental objectives:

1.   Become a healthy nation by promoting good health;
2.   Promote individual responsibility for one's own health and avoid overreliance on state welfare or third-party medical insurance;
3.   Ensure good and affordable basic medical services for all Singaporeans;
4.   Engage competition and market forces to improve service and raise efficiency; and
5.   Intervene directly in the healthcare sector when necessary, where the market fails to keep healthcare costs down.

Let us take a closer look at each of these objectives.

Promote Good Health

The White Paper set forth the need for health education, disease prevention, and motivating the population to adopt a healthy lifestyle and teaching the importance, for example, of leading an active life, not smoking, and eating the right foods in order to avoid obesity. To further these goals, the government created the Health Promotion Board (HPB). Its mission is to raise the level of health and health awareness through education, screening programs, dental services to children, nutrition programs, and more.

In effect, the government began to take the lead, working with agencies to reach out to groups within the population, developing an integrated and comprehensive approach. For example, the National Healthy Lifestyle campaign was given top political support.[24]

The National Healthy Lifestyle Campaign is an annual, month-long event that reaches into the community, workplace, schools, supermarkets, and restaurants. Healthy living themes are chosen—fighting obesity, for example—and activities such as mass workout sessions, weight loss reality television shows, school programs, and advertising are created around them. Some simple steps taken by the government to encourage healthy lifestyles include building exercise corners in all public housing, smooth pavements for people to walk and jog on, ensuring availability of healthier options at public food centers near public housing and transportation hubs, workplace health promotion programs, and the healthier choice symbol on foods.

The philosophy of healthy living is also evident today in nutrition counseling and nutrition support programs for patients in the hospitals, at outpatient clinics, and in the schools where the curriculum includes the basics of nutrition. Other programs are also available to the schools for promoting healthy eating habits among students.[25]

Promote Individual Responsibility for One's Own Health and Avoid Overreliance on State Welfare or Third-Party Medical Insurance

Singapore espouses the philosophy of individual responsibility: the population should be encouraged to cultivate a strong sense of personal responsibility toward health. The White Paper suggested that by making patients pay directly a part of their healthcare expenses, excessive demand for services could be mitigated and overreliance on state welfare or third-party medical insurance kept in check. It was asserted that the entitlement mentality—the notion that people are entitled to unlimited healthcare services at the expense of the state, employer, or an insurance company—should be prevented from gaining hold.

To avoid overreliance on comprehensive insurance programs that provided first-dollar coverage, the government incentivized the purchase of health insurance schemes with features such as deductible and co-payment components and guaranteed renewals by restricting the use of Medisave to only plans that met these requirements. Insurance plans that provided first-dollar coverage were viewed as playing a major role in raising costs in countries where they are readily available.

Administrative overheads alone, for example, are responsible for over 20 percent of the United States' total healthcare expenditure. It is thought that private insurance can also be responsible for over-consumption of care by patients, and over-delivery of services by doctors, as neither group is incentivized to keep costs in check as long as insurance companies will pay. Private insurance companies are also seen as discriminating against people at risk in favor of healthy individuals and so creating problems of equity, a condition that Singapore works very hard to avoid in its society.

Ensure Good and Affordable Basic Medical Services for All Singaporeans

In the White Paper, the government stated the need to make a good, basic medical package available to all people, whatever their means. The package did not necessarily have to make available the latest medical technologies but should include proven, cost-effective treatments, benefiting the maximum number of people. The package excluded certain treatments deemed not basic, such as cosmetic procedures and in-vitro fertilization (IVF, which is now subsidized, by the way.)

The basic package had to be affordable and be provided by hospitals receiving government subsidies. The most highly-subsidized ward classes were to offer this basic level of care.[26] The package should be reviewed frequently to reflect, among other things, the purchasing power of Singaporeans and productivity increases in medical science. In later years, means testing was initiated to ensure that government subsidies would be better targeted to help patients in greater financial need. Patients not meeting the criteria can still elect to go into the highly-subsidized wards, but they may not receive the maximum subsidy.

The White Paper foresaw that with the rising affluence of Singaporeans, the desire for sophisticated (and costly) medical services beyond the basic package would grow. It recommended that patients who were willing to spend more in order to obtain a different level of service be allowed to do so in the non-subsidized wards of public hospitals and in private hospitals.

In order to spur medical research, a plan was suggested under which the National University of Singapore (NUS) would focus on "academic research" that might provide valuable discoveries for the future. The subsidized hospitals were to focus on research that had "cost-effective" practical applications. The advancement of medical research in Singapore was furthered by the establishment in 1994 of the National Medical Research Council. It provides research funding to institutes and individuals, awards fellowships, and supports research that may one day be applied in medical practice, as well as clinical research.

Engage Competition and Market Forces to Improve Service and Raise Efficiency

The White Paper adopted the principle that resources available for healthcare were finite and must be put to efficient use. Market forces should be used to promote efficiency, improve quality of services, develop more choices for patients, and make sure patients are receiving good value for their money. It judged that healthcare providers were in a unique position to influence the demand for their services as patients rely on doctors for advice and are themselves generally unaware of better or competing alternatives. Yet, too much competition and too many providers might actually drive up the demand for medical services, since patients would naturally want to avail themselves to promising new treatments or technologies or popular doctors. Oversupply or overabundance of choices would in turn drive healthcare costs up rather than keep them in check and defeat the purpose of encouraging competition.

One step the Ministry of Health has taken to stoke competition is to provide price transparency by publishing the hospital bills for common illnesses on its website. One example of its effectiveness that I found striking is the drop in the price of LASIK surgery. In 2004, the price of the surgery for one eye was S$2,300. By 2008 the price had decreased to approximately S$1,400—a savings of S$1,000 per operation per eye.[27]

Intervene Directly in the Healthcare Sector, When Necessary, Where the Market Fails to Keep Healthcare Costs Down

I view Singapore's chosen approach to the healthcare market as a kind of highly-calibrated capitalism. Government intervention is sanctioned in certain circumstances to correct or redirect the market. This approach is seen in the fact that it funds public hospitals and other care facilities but also encourages the participation of private hospitals and clinics.

Situations that might demand government action included preventing an oversupply of healthcare services, moderating demand, and creating incentives to keep costs down. The White Paper also recommended that the government regulate specifics of the system. For example, over the years, intervention has included creating and adjusting medical savings programs, sponsoring insurance programs, providing subsidies to hospitals and polyclinics, determining the number of beds and their distribution in public hospitals, funding new medical schools, regulating the number and type of doctors who can practice in the country, and regulating and limiting the type and number of private insurance programs available to Singaporeans.

I will provide a closer look at a number of these practices for the development and maintenance of the system in subsequent chapters. But first, in the next chapter, I will walk you through the specific programs that make it possible for Singaporeans to pay for their care: Medisave and MediShield, as well as the safety net for those who cannot afford care: Medifund.

* * *

Chapter 1: KEY POINTS

- Singapore has built and maintains a high-quality healthcare system at a lower cost than any other high-income country in the world

- Four factors have enabled Singapore to achieve its remarkable health-care goals:

- ○ Political unity, constancy of purpose, and a culture of cooperation within government
- ○ Ability to recognize and establish national priorities, giving the economy time to grow before investing heavily in healthcare
- ○ An overwhelming desire for collective well-being and social harmony
- ○ Attention to the rights, education, and health needs of women

- Singapore's then Prime Minister Lee Kuan Yew envisioned a system that would not be "free" to consumers and would not contribute to a welfare state mentality nor diminish the people's desire to achieve and succeed

- Early actions to build the system included:
  - ○ Moving primary care to a network of outpatient clinics
  - ○ Charging patients for visits to clinics
  - ○ Sending doctors abroad to train in specialties
  - ○ Upgrading and updating care facilities
  - ○ Solving the housing crisis

- Singapore's National Health Care Plan, issued in 1983, set forth strategies for keeping care affordable and meeting the demands of a growing and increasingly affluent population. It also:
  - ○ Restructured the public hospital system, granting more autonomy to hospitals and promoting competition among them
  - ○ Introduced Medisave, a medical savings account that enabled individuals to put away money to pay for their healthcare

- The blueprint for Singapore's current healthcare system was published in 1993 as a White Paper entitled *Affordable Health Care*. It announced five objectives and set forth plans for implementing each:
  - ○ Become a healthy nation by promoting good health
  - ○ Promote individual responsibility for one's own health and avoid overreliance on state welfare or third-party medical insurance
  - ○ Ensure good and affordable basic medical services for all Singaporeans
  - ○ Engage competition and market forces to improve service and raise efficiency
  - ○ Intervene directly in the healthcare sector when necessary, where the market fails to keep healthcare costs down

CHAPTER 2

High Quality, Low Cost

Lee Kuan Yew wanted Singapore to achieve excellence—"first world standards" as he put it in his memoirs. Only then, he believed, would his young country survive and thrive. There is no doubt in my mind that the standards he desired for his city-state have indeed been met, and healthcare is one good example. Singapore now has a First-World healthcare system, rated sixth in the world by the World Health Organization and ahead of most high-income economies.[1] By most common measures, the nation has achieved noteworthy outcomes in all areas of healthcare. It has increased the life expectancy of its citizens; increased infant survival rates, and achieved one of the lowest under-five mortality rates in the world. Singapore's cancer survival rates are similar to Europe's, while its cardiovascular disease death rate is half that of the rest of the Asia Pacific region. As I will show throughout this chapter, Singapore produces world-class outcomes on par with the most-developed nations of the world, but it does so at a fraction of the cost usually associated with high-quality care.

A quick look at cost comparisons with other nations brings the point home. Countries like the United States and the United Kingdom struggle with the budget-busting, ever-rising cost increases of providing care. The United States, for example, spends almost 18 percent of GDP on healthcare. Singapore, on the other hand, spends slightly under four percent of GDP. The government's expenditure for healthcare has been slightly under one percent, far less than other most developed countries. It is, however, beginning to break the one percent barrier, coming in at just under 1.5 percent in 2010.[2]

I would like to begin our exploration of the Singapore healthcare system's achievements with a close-up look at some representative outcomes (see Table 2.1), how they have improved over the years, and how they compare with other nations in the region and around the world.

Table 2.1

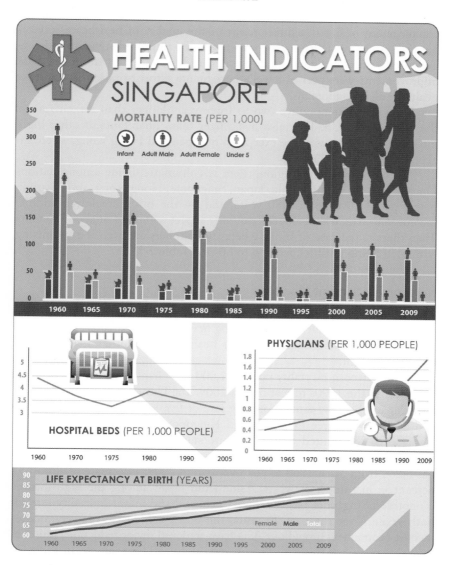

Life Expectancy

The number of years we may be expected to live is of utmost interest to all of us, and is a key measure of the efficacy of a nation's healthcare system. A Singaporean woman can now expect to live until 84, versus 66 in 1960. Singaporean men also live longer—up to 79 years, versus 62 in 1960. This enhancement of life is a direct result of the quality of healthcare services, but the system must share some credit with the improved standard of living, improved sanitation, good quality water, and a cleaner environment. Such improvements were part of a well-thought-out effort to raise the quality of health of all Singaporeans.

Singaporeans now live two to three years longer than the citizens of the UK and the US. They also live longer than inhabitants of other high-income economies, with the exception of Japan and Hong Kong, where life expectancy is up to 83 years.

In the Asia Pacific region, there is a dramatic divide among nations. On one side are countries like Japan, Singapore, Hong Kong, and Australia where people live beyond 80 years, and on the other are lower-middle-income countries where citizens can only expect a lifespan of about 70 years. Then there is the case of India, where the numbers are even less promising, with men living until 63, women to 66 (see Table 2.2).

Newborn and Infant Mortality

Another key measure of the success of Singapore's healthcare initiatives is the vastly improved survival rate among newborns and infants. A number of factors affect infant mortality, such as health of the mother, maternal care, and birth weight.

The newborn mortality rate per 1,000 live births in Singapore declined from five in the 1990s to just one in 2009. The United Kingdom, Australia, and Canada had the same mortality rate of five in the 1990s, but by 2009 had declined to three in the United Kingdom and Australia, and four in Canada. In the United States, the rate stands at four. Singapore's infant mortality rate (the probability of dying in the first year per 1,000 live births) has fallen from 36 in 1960 to just over two in 2009; a decrease of almost 94 percent in just under 50 years. Aside from Japan among the high-income economies, Singapore has the lowest neonatal and infant mortality rate for both sexes. Over the past 20 years, the upper-middle and lower-middle-income economies throughout Asia have achieved major reductions in infant mortality rates, but they still remain very high—50 for example, in India, 30 in Indonesia, 17 in China, and 12 in Vietnam (see Table 2.3).

Maternal mortality rates have also declined precipitously, from 86 deaths in 1950 to 12 deaths in 1975, to 3 in 2008.

Table 2.2

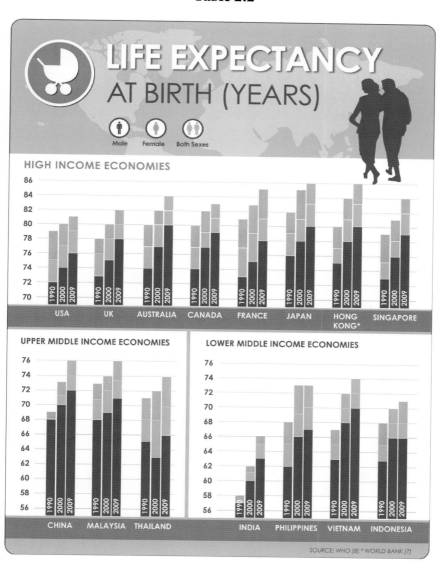

LIFE EXPECTANCY AT BIRTH (YEARS)

Male   Female   Both Sexes

HIGH INCOME ECONOMIES

USA   UK   AUSTRALIA   CANADA   FRANCE   JAPAN   HONG KONG*   SINGAPORE

UPPER MIDDLE INCOME ECONOMIES

CHINA   MALAYSIA   THAILAND

LOWER MIDDLE INCOME ECONOMIES

INDIA   PHILIPPINES   VIETNAM   INDONESIA

SOURCE: WHO [8].* WORLD BANK [7]

Table 2.3

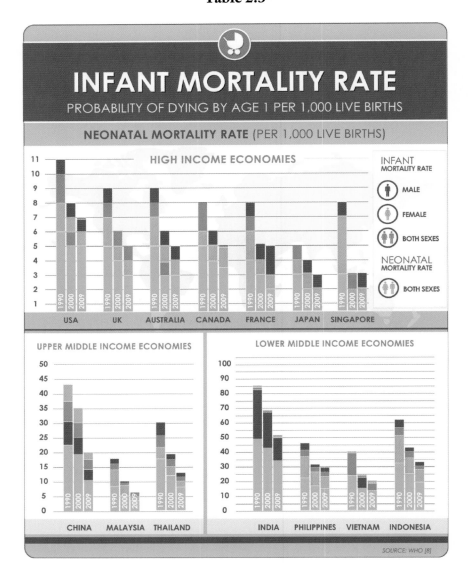

Under-Five Mortality Rate

This measure is an indication of the probability of dying by age five per 1,000 live births, and Singapore has achieved one of the lowest rates in the world. With ten deaths among men and eight among women in 1990, Singapore's current rate is three for men and two for women. Japan's numbers are similar, whereas the United States stands at eight for men and seven for women. The United Kingdom is at six for men and five for women. Under-five death rates are generally lower for women, even in the upper-middle and lower-middle-income countries with the exception of China and India. Within some countries, the disparities based on income are very large. For example, in India, children in the poorest 20 percent of the population are three times more likely to die before turning five as those in the richest 20 percent (see Table 2.4).

Childhood Diseases

Through the National Childhood Immunisation Programme, most childhood diseases have declined, with diphtheria, neonatal tetanus, poliomyelitis and congenital rubella virtually eliminated.[3]

Adult Mortality Rate

Singapore's adult mortality rate (defined as the probability of dying between the ages of 15 and 60 per 1,000 population) is significantly lower than the rest of Southeast Asia and even lower than developed countries. The rate has halved since 1990 and now stands at just under 60. The United States, by contrast, is just over 100 and Australia just over 60. Among the nations of Southeast Asia, there are very large variations in the rate—much greater than that observed for child mortality. Very high rates include India and Thailand at about 200 and China well over 100 (see Table 2.5).

Number of Physicians and Hospital Beds

Singapore performs well on other health indicators related to system infrastructure, including hospital beds available and physicians serving the population. A common measure of both is the number of beds or number of physicians (physician density) per 10,000 population. Another and perhaps more accurate way to find the ratio is to use the total number of beds in the acute sector in 2011 while excluding those in the Community Hospitals and the Chronic Sick Hospitals. Dividing the acute sector beds

Table 2.4

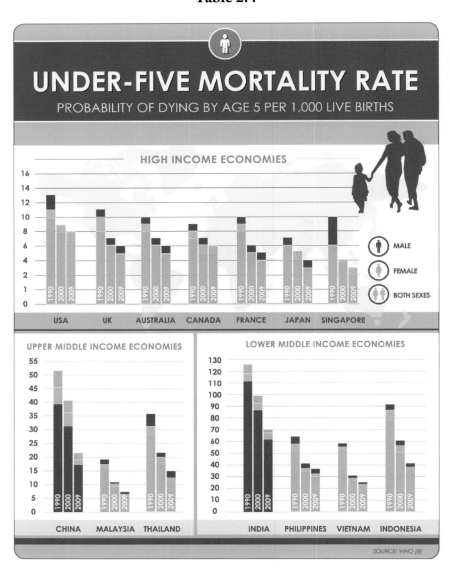

Table 2.5

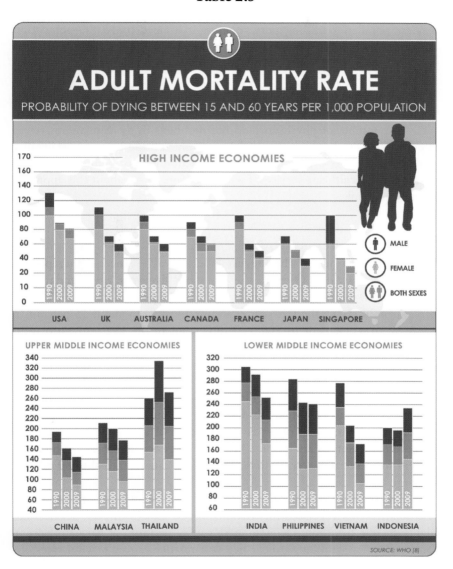

by the total Singapore population, we find a 1 bed-to-10,000-population ratio of about 20. Other developed countries have similar numbers, but Japan stands out with an extraordinary 140 beds. For Singapore, these numbers are derived from taking the total number of beds, including Community Hospital and Chronic Sick Hospital beds, and dividing by the resident population of Singapore, resulting in a 1 bed-to-10,000-population ratio of about 30.

Singapore is home to over 9,000 doctors according to the Singapore Medical Council, scoring a physician density rate of just over 18—higher than China, Malaysia, Thailand, and most other countries in the region, but behind the US and other high-income economies (see Table 2.6).

The number of physicians and hospital beds in the Singapore system is purposely kept in check to avoid oversupply and the too-easy availability of doctors or of beds. The idea behind this action is to prevent excessive and undue use of healthcare services. I will have more to say about this approach later in the book.

Cancer

With respect to one of the biggest killers of all—cancer—Singapore is making great strides. Overall, the country's five-year age standardized relative survival ratio for men improved from 14 percent in 1973–77 to 45 percent in 2003–07; the ten-year ratio improved from about 15 percent in 1978–82 to 41 percent in 2003–07. For women, the five-year ratio went from 28 to 58 percent during the same periods, and the 10-year numbers improved from 26 to 53 percent in those same 1973–77 and 2003–07 periods.[4]

While the Asia Pacific region contributes to half of all cancer deaths, survival is highest in Singapore, China, and South Korea with regard to cancers where prognosis depends on the stage of diagnosis. Survival rates in the three countries are in the 80 percent range for breast cancer, 60 to 80 percent for cervical cancer, 70 to 80 for bladder cancer, and 44 to 60 percent for large bowel cancers.[5]

One interesting comparison I found is that Singapore's one- and five-year relative survival ratios for nasopharyngeal cancer in both genders are higher than in the United Kingdom. Singapore performs at par with Europe for rectal, colon, and lung cancer five-year relative cancer survival rates, for cases diagnosed in 1995–99. And it performs better than Europe in stomach, liver (male five-year RSR), and ovarian cancer. Unfortunately, the county lags in bladder, corpus uteri, and female breast cancer survival rates.

Table 2.6

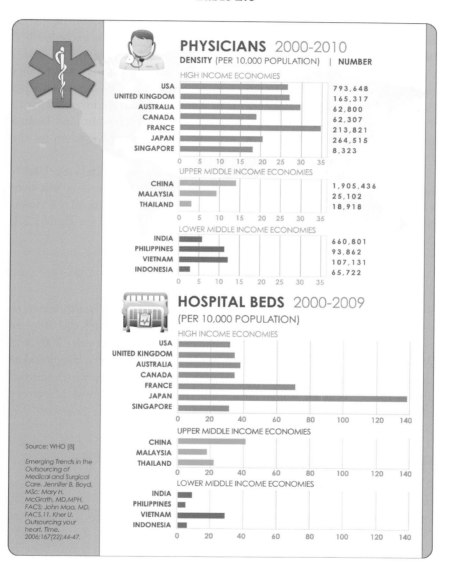

PHYSICIANS 2000-2010
DENSITY (PER 10,000 POPULATION) | **NUMBER**

HIGH INCOME ECONOMIES

Country	Number
USA	793,648
UNITED KINGDOM	165,317
AUSTRALIA	62,800
CANADA	62,307
FRANCE	213,821
JAPAN	264,515
SINGAPORE	8,323

UPPER MIDDLE INCOME ECONOMIES

Country	Number
CHINA	1,905,436
MALAYSIA	25,102
THAILAND	18,918

LOWER MIDDLE INCOME ECONOMIES

Country	Number
INDIA	660,801
PHILIPPINES	93,862
VIETNAM	107,131
INDONESIA	65,722

HOSPITAL BEDS 2000-2009
(PER 10,000 POPULATION)

HIGH INCOME ECONOMIES

USA
UNITED KINGDOM
AUSTRALIA
CANADA
FRANCE
JAPAN
SINGAPORE

UPPER MIDDLE INCOME ECONOMIES

CHINA
MALAYSIA
THAILAND

LOWER MIDDLE INCOME ECONOMIES

INDIA
PHILIPPINES
VIETNAM
INDONESIA

Source: WHO [8]

Emerging Trends in the
Outsourcing of
Medical and Surgical
Care. Jennifer B. Boyd,
MSc; Mary H.
McGrath, MD,MPH,
FACS; John Maa, MD,
FACS. 11. Kher U.
Outsourcing your
heart. Time.
2006;167(22):44-47.

Cardiovascular Disease

Cardiovascular disease is one of the main causes of deaths in developed countries. In the Asia Pacific region, the disease now accounts for as much as one-third of all deaths. In 2004, death rates in Japan, Australia, Singapore, and the Republic of Korea were lower than 200 per 100,000 people in contrast to the majority of countries in the region where it exceeded 400 deaths per 100,000.[6]

Singapore does not do quite as well with in-hospital case-fatality (within 30 days of admission) rates for acute myocardial infarction—with a rating of almost nine per 100 patients in 2007. Korea did slightly better with a rate of eight for the same year. Patients in United Kingdom and United States had lower fatality rates: just over six in the United Kingdom for the same year, and just over five in the United States in 2006.[7]

Ischemic stroke patients in Singapore had an in-hospital case-fatality rate of five, versus the United States' four (2006), and Korea's just over two. Korea attained a hemorrhagic stroke case-fatality rate of 11 versus Singapore's 25, with the United States at about 25 as well (see Figures 2.1, 2.2, and 2.3).

New Challenges

Singapore's success is also less clear in some of the newer health concerns arising among the populace. Diabetes is an example. Singapore's diabetes rate continues to rise, increasing by three percentage points between 2004 and 2010. As of 2010, over 11 percent of Singaporeans have been diagnosed as diabetic. This finding trends in parallel with increased obesity, which jumped almost four percentage points in the same time period to almost 11 percent of the population.[8]

Quality of Care

Not only does Singapore perform well in terms of achieving world-class outcomes, the quality of care as experienced by consumers is also one of the system's highest accomplishments. The Ministry of Health regularly conducts "Patient Satisfaction Surveys" to gauge the sentiments of the consumers of its health services. The seventh Patient Satisfaction Survey was done in 2010. It assessed the level of patient satisfaction, compared performance of the different healthcare institutions, and gathered feedback for service improvement. The survey found that over 75 percent of patients were satisfied

Figure 2.1

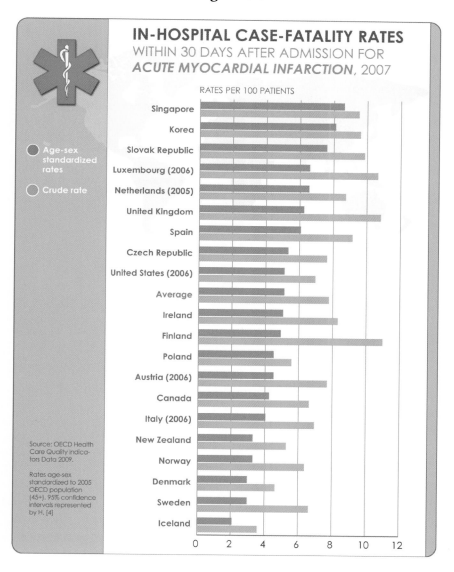

IN-HOSPITAL CASE-FATALITY RATES
WITHIN 30 DAYS AFTER ADMISSION FOR
ACUTE MYOCARDIAL INFARCTION, 2007

RATES PER 100 PATIENTS

Age-sex standardized rates

Crude rate

Singapore
Korea
Slovak Republic
Luxembourg (2006)
Netherlands (2005)
United Kingdom
Spain
Czech Republic
United States (2006)
Average
Ireland
Finland
Poland
Austria (2006)
Canada
Italy (2006)
New Zealand
Norway
Denmark
Sweden
Iceland

0   2   4   6   8   10   12

Source: OECD Health Care Quality Indicators Data 2009.

Rates age-sex standardized to 2005 OECD population (45+). 95% confidence intervals represented by H. [4]

Figure 2.2

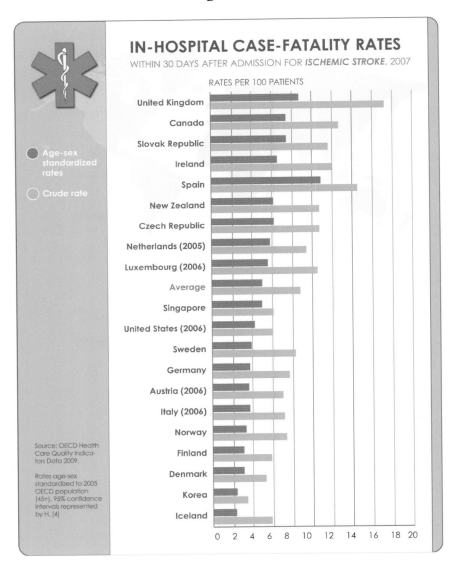

IN-HOSPITAL CASE-FATALITY RATES
WITHIN 30 DAYS AFTER ADMISSION FOR *ISCHEMIC STROKE*, 2007

RATES PER 100 PATIENTS

Age-sex standardized rates

Crude rate

United Kingdom
Canada
Slovak Republic
Ireland
Spain
New Zealand
Czech Republic
Netherlands (2005)
Luxembourg (2006)
Average
Singapore
United States (2006)
Sweden
Germany
Austria (2006)
Italy (2006)
Norway
Finland
Denmark
Korea
Iceland

0 2 4 6 8 10 12 14 16 18 20

Source: OECD Health Care Quality Indicators Data 2009.

Rates age-sex standardized to 2005 OECD population (45+). 95% confidence intervals represented by H. [4]

Figure 2.3

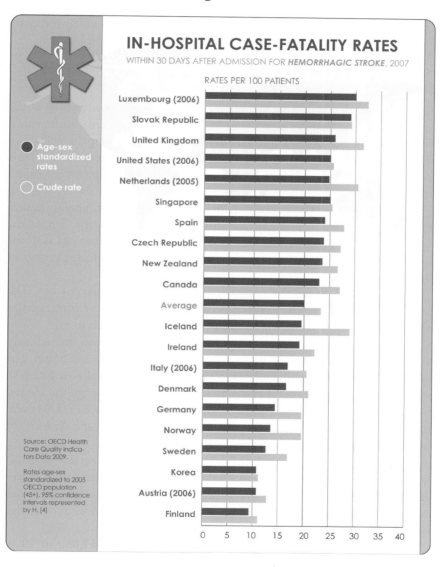

with the services at the public hospitals, polyclinics, and national specialty centers. Further, almost 80 percent would recommend the services of public healthcare institutions to others[9] (see Chart 2.1).

Confirming what Singapore's own self-assessments reveal, a World Health Organization report on comparative health systems issued in 2000 ranks Singapore's sixth globally in terms of overall performance. By comparison, the United States ranks 37, the United Kingdom 18, and Japan 10.[10]

Singapore's Healthcare Expenditure

Good healthcare is expensive, and many of the most-developed nations of the world are finding that the ever-rising costs for quality care are unsustainable. Singapore, on the other hand, has deftly managed to keep its costs low without sacrificing quality. In fact, it has achieved that exceptionally high rating from the World Health Organization while spending less per capita than any other high-income economy.

In spite of rising costs everywhere—due mainly to demographic trends, new and expensive technology, and changing disease patterns, Singapore, I am pleased to see, continues to spend less than four percent of GDP for healthcare, by far the lowest figure among all other high-income countries in the world.

The United States, by contrast, spends almost 18 percent of GDP annually—a huge price to pay that is currently causing bitter controversies and political battles as the nation debates its future approach to care.

When it comes to prices of specific procedures, one can immediately see the differences that exist in Singapore's costs vs. the United States. For example, the cost of an angioplasty in the United States is almost $83,000, while in Singapore the cost is about $13,000. A gastric bypass in the United States is almost US$70,000, while in Singapore the cost is $15,000 (these figures are in US dollars and include at least one day of hospitalization).[11] See Table 2.6a for more cost comparisons.

Singapore's total national health expenditure as a percentage of GDP is comparable to that of the upper-middle (China–Malaysia), and lower-middle-income countries (India–Philippines), but the health outcomes achieved are on par with those delivered by the highest-income countries in the world.

Singapore's per capita expenditure was just over US$2,000 in 2009. Comparison figures with other counties are available for 2008 and show that the United States spent the most per capita at just over US$7,000. Other developed countries on average spent over $3,000, except for Japan, which

Chart 2.1

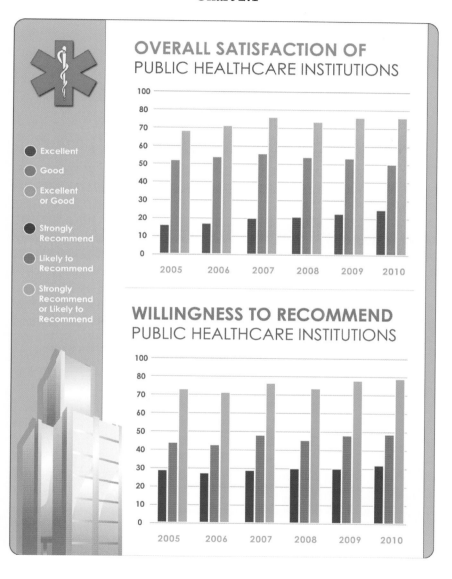

OVERALL SATISFACTION OF
PUBLIC HEALTHCARE INSTITUTIONS

Excellent
Good
Excellent or Good
Strongly Recommend
Likely to Recommend
Strongly Recommend or Likely to Recommend

2005 2006 2007 2008 2009 2010

WILLINGNESS TO RECOMMEND
PUBLIC HEALTHCARE INSTITUTIONS

2005 2006 2007 2008 2009 2010

Table 2.6a

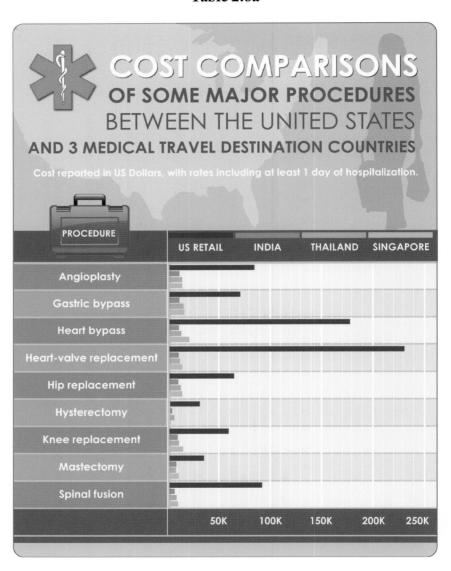

spent well under $3,000. In the lower-middle-income countries, the figure falls as low as $90, for example, in Indonesia. Singapore, in contrast, spent just over US$1,800.

Figures on government-only expenditure for the world's healthcare systems also show Singapore as the leader in keeping costs under control. Per capita studies reveal that in 2008, the government spent over $600 for care, while the United States spent almost $3,500, the United Kingdom over $2,600, Japan about $2,300. Asia Pacific figures range from $274 in Malaysia, $126 in China, down to $40. The Singapore government expenditure as a percentage of total government expenditure was around eight percent (see Tables 2.7, 2.8, and 2.8a).

Private expenditure in Singapore amounted to around 65 percent of the total national expense (2008). Note that this includes payments out of the government-run MediShield scheme and related insurance schemes, Medisave accounts, and other private insurance schemes or employer-provided medical benefits. The figure for the United States is 52 percent, 17 percent for the United Kingdom, and 18 percent Japan. Singapore's relatively high private expenditure is a direct result of the government's efforts to shift more of the cost burden to consumers than do most other countries. The approach is a fundamental strategy for keeping public expenditures down and curbing unnecessary usage. I would have to say that the approach is working. Later in the book, I will take a much closer look at this strategy, as well as the system's guiding principle of encouraging individuals' responsibility for their own care.

I find it interesting that the figures for private healthcare expenditure in lower-middle-income countries are also substantial, but for a different reason. The underdeveloped public healthcare infrastructure in these countries and a general lack of faith in the system cause citizens to gravitate toward private healthcare services and to pay for their own care. In India, private expenditure was as high as 67 percent in 2008; in the Philippines it amounted to around 65 percent.

Singapore's Advantages

Along with its excellent system of medical care, Singapore has developed an infrastructure that helps support healthy living and general wellness: an inexpensive and affordable mass transit system, neighborhood wet markets (fresh food markets) and supermarkets that carry affordable fresh fruit and vegetables, islandwide park connectors and HDB exercise stations, Ministry-funded community centers in every neighborhood, and close proximity to family and other support systems.

Table 2.7

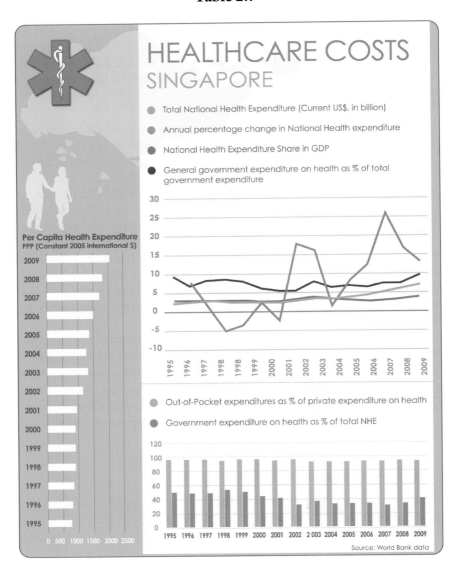

HEALTHCARE COSTS
SINGAPORE

- Total National Health Expenditure (Current US$, in billion)
- Annual percentage change in National Health expenditure
- National Health Expenditure Share in GDP
- General government expenditure on health as % of total government expenditure

Per Capita Health Expenditure
PPP (Constant 2005 international $)

- Out-of-Pocket expenditures as % of private expenditure on health
- Government expenditure on health as % of total NHE

Source: World Bank data

Table 2.8

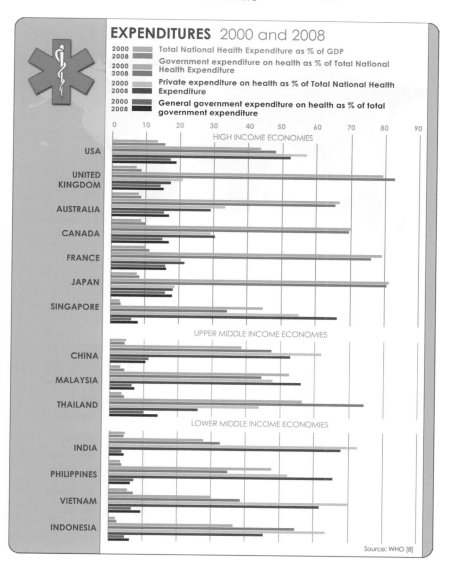

EXPENDITURES 2000 and 2008

- 2000 / 2008 — Total National Health Expenditure as % of GDP
- 2000 / 2008 — Government expenditure on health as % of Total National Health Expenditure
- 2000 / 2008 — Private expenditure on health as % of Total National Health Expenditure
- 2000 / 2008 — General government expenditure on health as % of total government expenditure

HIGH INCOME ECONOMIES

USA
UNITED KINGDOM
AUSTRALIA
CANADA
FRANCE
JAPAN
SINGAPORE

UPPER MIDDLE INCOME ECONOMIES

CHINA
MALAYSIA
THAILAND

LOWER MIDDLE INCOME ECONOMIES

INDIA
PHILIPPINES
VIETNAM
INDONESIA

Source: WHO [8]

Table 2.8a

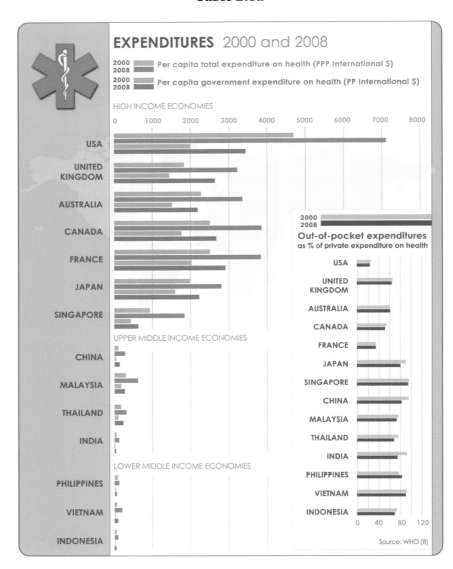

In addition, Singapore's economy and environment have played a role in its healthcare achievement. The country's wealth, high employment rate, compactness and lack of rural areas, and relatively low number of immigrants give it some advantages in its continuing efforts to nurture and sustain the excellence of its system.

Singapore's government leaders, ministers, and care professionals have developed a healthcare system with some of the best outcomes in the world, and as I have explained, with far less cost to the economy than might reasonably be expected. In the following chapters, I will explore how exactly they accomplished this extraordinary feat.

* * *

Chapter 2: KEY POINTS

- Singapore's healthcare system has achieved First World standards at a lower cost than any high-income country in the world

- The system has achieved excellent outcomes by most common measures:
  - Increased life expectancy of its citizens
  - Increased infant survival rates
  - One of the lowest under-five mortality rates in the world
  - An adult mortality rate lower than any nation's
  - Hospital beds ratios similar to the United States'
  - Cancer survival rates similar to Europe's
  - Cardiovascular disease death rates half of most countries in the region

- Singapore's quality of care is excellent:
  - Most consumers of its services report a high level of satisfaction
  - It is ranked sixth in the world by the World Health Organization

- Cost of care has been kept low while achieving very high quality:
  - It spends less per capita than any other high-income nation
  - The government outlays per capita for the system are a fraction of what developed nations spend
  - Private expenditure is relatively high compared to many countries, in keeping with the government philosophy that people must be responsible for their own care

Helping Patients Pay

The success of healthcare in Singapore today is largely due to the government's creative use of the Central Provident Fund. The CPF's medical savings component, called Medisave, makes it possible for Singaporeans to pay for much of their own medical care. Medisave is, in essence, a compulsory savings account. The government sets contribution rates for workers and their employers as a percentage of wages. Once in their accounts, the money may be used to pay for personal and family healthcare—always along carefully-established guidelines.

As mentioned in Chapter 1, the Central Provident Fund was first introduced under British colonial rule and functioned as a simple, mandatory retirement savings plan. Workers contributed five percent of their wages into the Fund, and their employers matched the amount.[1] The nest eggs grew through these combined contributions plus interest paid on the balances. When participants reached 55, people could begin withdrawing the money to help pay for retirement.

Soon after independence, the government expanded the scope of the CPF and turned it into a vital factor in improving the lives, living conditions, and health of Singaporeans. It was determined early on that compelling health savings would play an increasingly larger role in the lives of the people, and it became a central part of long-term planning. Changes to the Fund were to be introduced in small doses over the years, so as not to cause concern and confusion among the population and to make them more acceptable. As wages rose, so too did the percentage of the salary contribution to the CPF. However, the increases were carefully calibrated so that an increase in wages always meant a net increase in take-home pay.[2]

The first significant step was taken in 1968 when, for the first time, in addition to retirement expenses, workers were allowed to use a portion of their CPF to help purchase apartments built by the Housing and Development Board. Since then, the rules governing the Fund have been changed to allow workers to use their savings to also pay for healthcare, approved insurance schemes, and education.

When employed Singaporeans and their employers make their monthly contributions, the money is dispersed into three accounts: Ordinary Account: to be used to buy a home, pay for CPF insurance against death and disability, investment and education; Special Account: for old age and investment in retirement-related financial products; and Medisave Account: to be used for healthcare expenses and approved medical insurance.

The mandatory allocation among the three accounts changes according to the age of the participant. 30-year-olds see their total contribution divided as follows: 23 percent of wages to the Ordinary Account; six percent to the Special Account; and seven percent to Medisave. For 50-year-olds: 19 percent to Ordinary; eight percent to Special; nine percent to Medisave. The "percent of wage" figures represent the combined contribution of employee and employer.

I will focus on the Fund's healthcare components and the central role they play in maintaining the health and wellness of Singaporeans. The component parts that impact healthcare include: medical care savings programs (Medisave); supplemental catastrophic, chronic, and long-term care insurance programs (MediShield); as well as funds for paying healthcare costs for the poor (Medifund). Together, they are known as the 3Ms—Medisave, MediShield, and Medifund—and I believe they play an integral role in the success of the system. Private insurance plays a limited role, and I will examine it as well.

What Patients Pay For

The government provides access to a basic level of care and subsidizes most of its cost so that no one goes without fundamental healthcare. However, as I have discussed, the system is designed to make sure patients do contribute to the cost of their care. In addition, as part of the system's choice initiative, patients are allowed to spend their own money on care beyond the basic level, including amenities in public hospitals, private hospitals, private doctors, and other services. They pay the costs using their own money, Medisave funds, and approved health insurance within the limitations established by guidelines, which I will explain in this chapter. No one, then, is obligated to stay with the publicly subsidized programs if they are willing to pay for some things beyond what they offer.

Table 3.1

CPF CONTRIBUTION & ALLOCATION
RATES FOR THE VARIOUS TYPES OF EMPLOYEES

FOR:

(1) PRIVATE SECTOR,

(2) NON-PENSIONABLE EMPLOYEES (STATUTORY BODIES & AIDED SCHOOLS),

(3) NON-PENSIONABLE EMPLOYEES (MINISTRIES)

NOTE: FOR (1), (2) AND (3), THE ORDINARY WAGE CEILING IS $5,000.

CONTRIBUTION RATE
For monthly wages exceeding $1,500

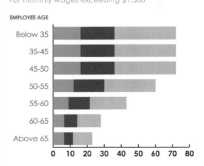
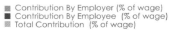

CREDITED INTO

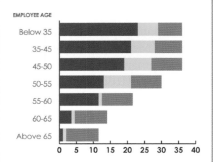

- ■ Contribution By Employer (% of wage)
- ■ Contribution By Employee (% of wage)
- ▨ Total Contribution (% of wage)

- ■ Ordinary Account(% of wage)
- ▨ Special Account(% of wage)
- ■ MEDISAVE Account(% of wage)

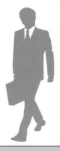

(a) Singapore Citizen

(b) SPR in the 3rd year and onwards of obtaining SPR status,

(c) SPR in the 1st and 2nd year of obtaining SPR status but who has jointly applied with employer to contribute at full employer and employee rates

Note: If the monthly wages are less than $1,500, please refer to the CPF Contribution Rates Table.

Table 3.1a

CPF CONTRIBUTION & ALLOCATION
RATES FOR THE VARIOUS TYPES OF EMPLOYEES

FOR:

(1) PENSIONABLE EMPLOYEES (Statutory Bodies)

(2) PENSIONABLE EMPLOYEES (Ministries)

NOTE: FOR (1) and (2), THE ORDINARY WAGE CEILING IS $6,666.67.

CONTRIBUTION RATE
For monthly wages exceeding $1,500

CREDITED INTO

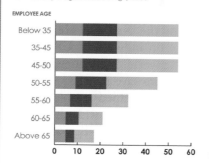

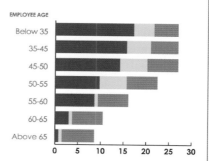

- ■ Contribution By Employer (% of wage)
- ■ Contribution By Employee (% of wage)
- ■ Total Contribution (% of wage)

- ■ Ordinary Account (% of wage)
- Special Account (% of wage)
- ■ MEDISAVE Account (% of wage)

(a) Singapore Citizen

(b) SPR in the 3rd year and onwards of obtaining SPR status,

(c) SPR in the 1st and 2nd year of obtaining SPR status but who has jointly applied with employer to contribute at full employer and employee rates

The public hospitals provide a good example of how the system works. Wards are classified by amenities and level of government subsidy provided. There are five ward classes: A, B1, B2+, B2, and C. A costs the patient most, and C the least. A-class patients have a private room with a bathroom, air conditioning, and access to private doctors of their choice. C-class patients are in open wards, eight to nine in a room, sharing a bathroom, and without air conditioning. Their doctors are assigned to them.

There is no government subsidy for A-class patients, while those in C-class receive a subsidy of up to 80 percent of inpatient ward charges, drugs, and other medical treatment. C-class patients also receive subsidies on surgical procedures and on physicians' fees. In all the other wards between A and C, amenities and choices decline as the subsidy increases. Financial means testing is used to determine eligibility for subsidy for anyone seeking admittance to C and B2 wards. I will provide more details on all this in a later chapter.[3]

Medisave

Medisave was the first health-related expansion of the Central Provident Fund. Initially unveiled in 1983 as part of the National Health Plan, Medisave was created as an account within an individual's CPF. At the time, Medisave was the first of its kind in the world. It contained a simple and powerful idea: help the people of Singapore save for their healthcare expenses, just as the Central Provident Fund helped people save for retirement. I view Medisave as an initiative in keeping with the national philosophy encouraging self-reliance, personal responsibility, and family responsibility. Since it was determined by the architects of the system early on that individuals would pay for most of their healthcare cost after heavy government subsidy, the government saw Medisave as a way to ensure everyone would have money to do so.

Contributions to Medisave

Under Medisave, workers and their employers contribute a specified percentage of monthly wages to the individual's CPF account of which a certain portion, as I pointed out above, goes into Medisave. Contributions are based on the age of the employee. As of 2012, workers up through age 50 contribute 20 percent of their wages, and their employers add another 16 percent for a total contribution equaling 36 percent of their wages. The money is divided into the three abovementioned accounts, with the Medisave account receiving between 7 and 9.5 percent of the wage depending on age. The worker contribution is lowered to 18.5 percent for those over 50 through 55, and the employer rate drops to 14 percent, with 9.5 percent going to Medisave. Above age 65, employee contribution drops to five percent, employers 6.5 percent, with 9.5 percent of wage going to Medisave (see Table 3.1). This is not considered to be a tax by the Singaporeans I have met, no more than are the 401k plans of the United States.

All the savings are tax exempt, both at the time of deposit and of withdrawal, and they are guaranteed to earn a fixed interest rate established by the CPF Board with a minimum rate of 2.5 percent. In recent years, the rate had stayed at 4 percent. The rate is often pegged to the average yield of specifically-designated Singapore Government Securities. Self-employed individuals initially were excluded from Medisave, but beginning in 1992, anyone earning above S$6,000 a month was also required to contribute. The self-employed must declare their income to the government and from there a determination is made on the amount of their Medisave contribution.

The government sets a maximum amount that individuals can accumulate in their Medisave account. The maximum specified for Medisave is presumed to be adequate for an individual's projected future healthcare needs, freeing up the person's other funds to go toward other retirement purposes. In 2012, it was fixed at S$43,500, but the ceiling is adjusted yearly to take into account the impact of healthcare inflation and to ensure that account holders have sufficient savings by the time of retirement. Contributions beyond the ceiling are transferred to other CPF accounts.[4]

The government also sets account minimums; this is the amount individuals must retain in their Medisave accounts when they make a withdrawal of CPF savings. In 2012, it required participants 55 and over to have at least S$32,000 in their accounts. If that minimum is not met, then the account must be topped-up before withdrawals from excess savings in other CPF accounts will be allowed. Account holders need to name a beneficiary to whom the funds are passed upon death, or the funds will be distributed in accordance with intestacy laws.

Putting Medisave Funds to Use

Although dollars put into a Medisave account belong to the contributing worker, the government has issued tight guidelines over how the money can be spent. But as part of an ongoing task, it remains responsive to the healthcare environment and continually revises the guidelines on how funds can be used as conditions change. All this while keeping to its principle of balancing affordable healthcare against over-consumption and preventing the premature depletion of Medisave funds.

A Singaporean may use his Medisave to pay for certain medical expenses. Immediate family members (spouse, parents, and children) are allowed to draw upon each other's accounts. Initially, Medisave could only be used to pay for charges for a hospital stay in the highly-subsidized wards. Gradually it was extended to include other hospital ward classes but subject to maximum daily limits. Now it can be used to pay for hospitalization charges as well as specified outpatient expenses. Medisave can presently be used for medical and surgical inpatient cases, approved day surgeries, and psychiatry treatment. Stays in approved community hospitals, hospices, maternity, and day rehabilitation are also eligible. Also allowed are treatment in approved day hospitals, outpatient treatments of approved chronic diseases, vaccinations, outpatient MRI scans, CT scans and other diagnostics for cancer patients, assisted conception procedures, and renal dialysis treatment. Cancer patients may use Medisave for radiotherapy, radio surgery, and chemotherapy. Also eligible are HIV anti-retroviral drugs, desferal drug and blood transfusion for Thalassemia treatment, hyperbaric oxygen therapy, outpatient intravenous antibiotic treatment, long-term oxygen therapy and infant continuous positive airway pressure therapy, immune-suppressants for patients after organ transplants.[5] Medisave and insurance do not cover the costs of consultation alone. Patients generally pay out of pocket if they wish to seek a second opinion.

Recent guideline changes have reflected the changing demographics of the nation and the changing needs of the populace, as well as voter sentiment. Some examples:

Women 50 and over may spend up to S$400 from their Medisave for mammogram screening. The usual cost at polyclinics is S$100. However, the test is offered at a subsidized rate of S$50 for citizens and S$75 for permanent residents.[6] To address the increase in chronic diseases as Singapore's proportion of elderly people grows, a new program helps pay for outpatient treatment of common chronic conditions: diabetes mellitus, hypertension, lipid disorders, stroke, asthma, chronic obstructive pulmonary disorder, schizophrenia, major depression, bipolar disorder, and dementia. The program provides incentives for people to seek structured treatment and management of their chronic diseases at the primary care level, where better disease management can help reduce the need for hospitalization. A S$30 deductible and a co-payment of 15 percent of the total bill still needs to be paid by the individual, but Medisave can be used to pay the remaining balance of the bill. Up to ten family-related accounts can be drawn upon, and the annual withdrawal limit is capped at S$400 per year for each account.[7]

In Singapore, the birthrate has been well below replacement levels for many years, a matter of great concern for the future of the country. The total fertility rate in 2011 was just over one child per woman. A rate of two children per woman is considered necessary to keep the population at current levels. Rates below two children indicate that the population is decreasing with a growing percentage of older people.[8] Furthermore, Singaporeans are marrying later, having children later, or choosing to have fewer children.[9]

In a demonstration of the system's willingness to respond to the financial and healthcare needs of its current citizens, as well as the state's own need to increase the numbers of its future citizens, the government has introduced a number of programs. Among them: the government has extended the use of Medisave dollars to fertility treatments as well as to maternity care. Medisave can now be used to pay for delivery expenses as well as pre-delivery medical expenses. Up to S$450 can be withdrawn for each day of the hospital stay, an additional amount for the delivery procedure itself, as well as an additional S$450 for pre-delivery medical expenses. Payments for assisted conception procedures are also allowed: S$6,000, S$5,000, and S$4,000 can be withdrawn for the first, second, and third claims respectively (see Table 3.2).[10]

MediShield will for the first time cover congenital and neonatal conditions, and newborns will have a government-paid S$3,000 Medisave account.[11]

The Marriage and Parenthood Package 2013, a S$2billion/year program, has also been introduced to encourage childbearing. Components include a baby bonus—a cash gift given to married couples on the birth of each of their children. Couples receive S$6,000 for each of the first and second children, and S$8,000 for each of the third and fourth children. Additionally, the couple may open a savings account, called a Child Development Account, for each of their children. Parents may contribute to the account and receive dollar-for-dollar matched donations from the government capped at S$6,000 each for the first and second children, S$12,000 for the third and fourth children, and S$18,000 for each subsequent child. The savings may be used to pay for approved early childhood education and healthcare expenses.[12]

Most childhood vaccinations are free-of-charge, while vaccinations for Hepatitis B, Pneumococcal disease, and the human papillomavirus are not. But Medisave can be used to pay for all three and no co-payment or deductible is required.[13]

Table 3.2

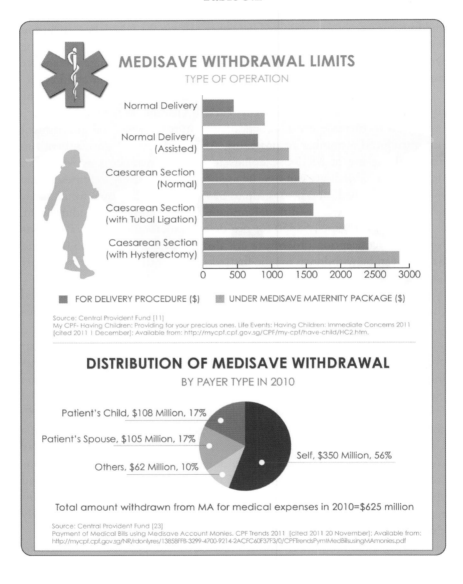

MEDISAVE WITHDRAWAL LIMITS
TYPE OF OPERATION

Normal Delivery

Normal Delivery (Assisted)

Caesarean Section (Normal)

Caesarean Section (with Tubal Ligation)

Caesarean Section (with Hysterectomy)

0   500   1000   1500   2000   2500   3000

■ FOR DELIVERY PROCEDURE ($)   ■ UNDER MEDISAVE MATERNITY PACKAGE ($)

Source: Central Provident Fund [11]
My CPF- Having Children: Providing for your precious ones. Life Events: Having Children: Immediate Concerns 2011 [cited 2011 1 December]; Available from: http://mycpf.cpf.gov.sg/CPF/my-cpf/have-child/HC2.htm.

DISTRIBUTION OF MEDISAVE WITHDRAWAL
BY PAYER TYPE IN 2010

Patient's Child, $108 Million, 17%

Patient's Spouse, $105 Million, 17%

Others, $62 Million, 10%

Self, $350 Million, 56%

Total amount withdrawn from MA for medical expenses in 2010=$625 million

Source: Central Provident Fund [23]
Payment of Medical Bills using Medisave Account Monies. CPF Trends 2011 [cited 2011 20 November]; Available from: http://mycpf.cpf.gov.sg/NR/rdonlyres/13858FFB-3299-4700-9214-2ACFC60F37F3/0/CPFTrendsPymtMedBillsusingMAmonies.pdf

Sharing Medisave among Family Members

Medisave was designed to allow families to share the benefits of the program as well as the burden of healthcare costs, allowing families to pool risks amongst themselves. Statistics from 2010 show that family members are taking good advantage of the plan and are making use of accumulated dollars in each others' accounts. According to the CPF Board, about one million medical bills were paid in 2010, and about S$625 million were withdrawn from Medisave accounts to pay those bills. 56 percent of the total dollars came from patients' own accounts, while the remainder was taken from the accounts of patients' children, spouses, parents, and grandchildren. Patients younger than 55 tended to draw principally from their own accounts and from their spouses', while older patients used their own accounts and those of their children (see Chart 3.1).

Government Contributions to Medisave

Another example of the government's responsiveness to changing conditions is that from time to time it provides grants or "top ups" directly into Singaporeans' Medisave accounts.

In the 2011 budget, a "Grow and Share Package" was announced with the declared intention of sharing the nation's prosperity with the people by contributing money to their Medisave accounts. The plan principally benefited lower and middle-income citizens, and only those aged 45 and above. Annual income and the value of the individual's home were taken into consideration to determine the amount to be received. It was estimated that the majority of Singaporeans would be given from S$200 to S$700 each. This measure would aid well over one million Singaporeans and cost the government about S$500 million (see Table 3.3).[14]

Since 2007, the government also provides regular annual Medisave top-ups under the Workfare Income Supplement scheme, a permanent scheme to supplement the wages and CPF savings of older low-wage workers. In the 2012 budget, the government further introduced additional assistance for low-income Singaporeans through the GST Voucher Scheme which helps to offset up to half of the GST paid each year. The assistance includes an annual Medisave top-up ranging from S$150 to S$450 to help low-income elderly Singaporeans aged 65 and above with their healthcare expenses.[15]

Self-employed persons were also given some benefit in the package. Tax deductions were granted to eligible companies that made voluntary contributions to the Medisave account of employees, capped at S$1,500 per person per year. No tax would be due from the recipients (see Table 3.4). The

Chart 3.1

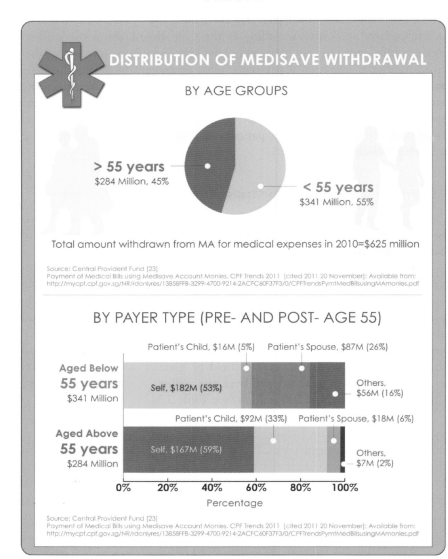

DISTRIBUTION OF MEDISAVE WITHDRAWAL

BY AGE GROUPS

> 55 years
$284 Million, 45%

< 55 years
$341 Million, 55%

Total amount withdrawn from MA for medical expenses in 2010=$625 million

Source: Central Provident Fund [23]
Payment of Medical Bills using Medisave Account Monies. CPF Trends 2011 [cited 2011 20 November]; Available from:
http://mycpf.cpf.gov.sg/NR/rdonlyres/13858FFB-3299-4700-9214-2ACFC60F37F3/0/CPFTrendsPymtMedBillsusingMAmonies.pdf

BY PAYER TYPE (PRE- AND POST- AGE 55)

Patient's Child, $16M (5%)   Patient's Spouse, $87M (26%)

**Aged Below
55 years**
$341 Million

Self, $182M (53%)

Others,
$56M (16%)

Patient's Child, $92M (33%)   Patient's Spouse, $18M (6%)

**Aged Above
55 years**
$284 Million

Self, $167M (59%)

Others,
$7M (2%)

0%   20%   40%   60%   80%   100%

Percentage

Source: Central Provident Fund [23]
Payment of Medical Bills using Medisave Account Monies. CPF Trends 2011 [cited 2011 20 November]; Available from:
http://mycpf.cpf.gov.sg/NR/rdonlyres/13858FFB-3299-4700-9214-2ACFC60F37F3/0/CPFTrendsPymtMedBillsusingMAmonies.pdf

Table 3.3

TOP UP FOR CPF MEDISAVE ACCOUNT

ASSESSABLE INCOME for YA 2010	ANNUAL VALUE OF RESIDENCE (As at 31 December 2010) Up to $7,000

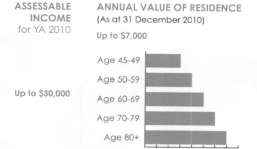

ASSESSABLE INCOME for YA 2010	ANNUAL VALUE OF RESIDENCE (As at 31 December 2010) More Than $7,000

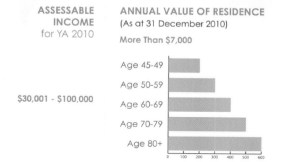

Source: Singapore Budget 2011 [25]
Singapore Budget 2011: Benefits for Households.
Singapore Budget: Key Budget Initiatives [cited 2011 2 December];
Available from: http://www.mof.gov.sg/budget_2011/key_initiatives/families.html - s2

Table 3.4

TAX BENEFITS
FOR VOLUNTARY CONTRIBUTIONS
by Companies to Self-Employed Persons' Medisave Account

CURRENT TREATMENT

For Self-Employed Persons:

Medisave contributions made by eligible Companies to the Self-Employed individuals' CPF accounts may be considered taxable income.

NEW TREATMENT

For Self-Employed Persons:

Medisave contributions made by eligible Companies to Self-Employed individuals' Medisave account will now be tax-exempt up to a cap of $1,500 for each calendar year.

The limit will remain at $1,500 for Self-Employed Persons with more than one Company.

CURRENT TREATMENT

For Companies:

Companies who voluntarily contribute to Self-Employed individuals' CPF accounts are not given tax deductions.

1. In addition, the Medisave contributions have to be within the CPF Annual Limit of the recipient and Medisave Contribution Ceiling prevailing at the point of contribution.

2. Employers can contribute to their Employee's Medisave account to obtain tax deductions of up to $1,500 through the Additional Medisave Contribution Scheme.

Source: Central Provident Fund [26] Singapore Budget 2011: Initiatives Relating to CPF, General Information: Singapore Budget 2011: Initiatives Relating to CPF 2011 [cited 2011 10 November]. Available from: http://mycpf.cpf.gov.sg/Members/Genlnfo/CPFChanges/Budget2011_CPF.htm.

NEW TREATMENT

For Companies:

Eligible Companies who voluntarily contribute to Self-Employed individuals' Medisave account will be allowed tax deductions up to $1,500 per Self-Employed for each calendar year.

For Self-Employed Persons with more than one Company, the $1,500 tax deduction will be apportioned between the Companies in the order in which their contributions were made.

For members who are both Self-Employed and an Employee, the $1,500 tax deduction will be apportioned between the Company and Employer for eligible top-ups in the order in which their contributions were made.

government has made it clear, however, that measures such as the Medisave top up are undertaken at its own volition and should not be considered a right of citizens or an ongoing obligation of the government. Individuals must continue to be responsible for their own health and their own health-care costs.

Medisave's Effect on the System

There is little doubt that the manner in which medical care is paid for has an impact on costs. Singapore has countered rising healthcare costs to a far greater degree than in all other high-income countries. Perhaps when people have to spend their own money, as the Singapore system requires, they tend to be more economical in the solutions they pursue for their medical problems. In contrast, in countries with third-party reimbursement systems, neither providers nor consumers of healthcare bear the major burden of cost. Since someone else is paying—government programs, insurance companies— there is little incentive to be prudent in decisions about which and how many tests and treatments are appropriate for a given situation.

I see Medisave as central to providing citizens a quality of life com-parable to the most affluent nations of the world, despite the poverty and adverse conditions that existed in Singapore in its earliest days of independence. By keeping costs down, Medisave has allowed the entire system to remain more affordable to everyone, including the government. A survey published in 2008 showed that people had a high level of confidence in the healthcare system and agreed that care was generally affordable, especially at the polyclinics and public-sector hospitals. There was some growing concern, however, that tertiary care—specialty care—was less affordable.[16]

Some, however, disagree with this assessment that gives credit to the system of medical savings accounts for the success of the Singapore healthcare system. One critic has a rather harsh view of the system, saying that "the heart of the Singapore system of health funding, with its financial discipline, is government control of inputs and outputs and strict rationing of health services according to wealth."[17] It is necessary to examine this kind of criticism in order to find and eliminate flaws even in a system as laudable as Singapore's.

Medisave has allowed the government to focus assistance programs on the very needy who are unable to pay for their own care. I will be examining one such program—Medifund—later in the chapter. Medisave has been successful in helping people pay for their care and for keeping the cost of care within bounds. I wish I could say that is the end of the story. Unfortunately, it is not. Costs keep rising, families keep getting smaller, limiting the ability to share Medisave dollars, and people are living longer and needing more care. The government, to its credit, saw these problems unfolding and decided the people of Singapore needed more help paying bills, especially when major, potentially financially-ruinous illnesses struck. Thus, a new component—the second M—was added to the Central Provident Fund, and that is catastrophic health insurance.

Interestingly, China has exported some of the basic ideas behind the medical savings accounts for use in Shanghai. Unfortunately, according to one study, the experiment has not been a success. According to the author, "With no sufficient safety net and no alternative healthcare coverage, a large proportion of Shanghai residents are facing uncertainty. One person's major illness can cause his/her family a disastrous financial burden." Without Singapore's wealth, its relatively younger population, its higher employment rate, its lack of rural areas, and its limited number of immigrants, Shanghai has not been able to emulate the effectiveness of Singapore's use of medical savings accounts.[18]

MediShield—Insuring Against Catastrophic Illness

MediShield is a low-cost medical insurance scheme created in 1990, six years after Medisave, and available to CPF members and their dependents. The idea behind MediShield is to provide assistance to individuals with prolonged illnesses that may require long-term medical treatment—treatment that can become very expensive over time and a burden on families, possibly draining their Medisave accounts. MediShield, under designated circumstances, helps cover a portion of expenses for hospitalization and certain outpatient treatments, such as kidney dialysis and approved cancer treatments, such as chemotherapy and radiotherapy.

Individuals are automatically insured under MediShield unless they specifically choose to opt out, and over 90 percent of the population is insured. The government will do more to raise this percentage further.

CPF members can insure themselves and their dependents under MediShield if the dependants are citizens or permanent residents—up to 85 years of age.

As a catastrophic health insurance, MediShield focuses its benefits on helping patients pay for treatment of very serious illnesses or for prolonged hospitalization in subsidized wards (Class C and B2) of public hospitals—those providing subsidies of up to 80 percent to Singapore citizens.[19]

Annual premiums for MediShield are not expensive, and Medisave funds can be used to pay for them. For example, a 29-year-old pays only S$33 yearly; a 49-year-old pays S$114; a 69-year-old pays S$372 (see Table 3.5). After the end of each policy year, MediShield coverage is automatically renewed after the premium has been paid from a Medisave account.

Enrollment must take place before the age of 75. The maximum claim limit per policy year is S$50,000, with a S$200,000 lifetime cap. There is some concern that the caps are inadequate, and it is possible that they will be raised. Additionally, the Ministry of Health is discussing other changes, including extending coverage to people with congenital conditions.[20]

According to the Ministry, members wishing to have more coverage are free to purchase Medisave-approved Integrated Shield plans through which individuals' needs can be addressed. They are also free to purchase additional non-Medisave-approved policies to cover the deductibles and co-insurance, though individuals must pay cash for these plans.[21]

In keeping with the philosophy that patients must bear responsibility for their healthcare, MediShield is not designed to pick up all costs. A ceiling is imposed—known as the claimable limit—on the amount that can be reimbursed for any given bill. The ceiling is determined by established maximum limits per day of hospitalization, surgical procedures, surgical implants, and specific treatments.

An annual deductible against claims must be met and "co-insurance" must be paid before MediShield coverage can begin, but Medisave dollars or cash can be used to pay these first obligations. Co-insurance is the percentage of the bill patients pay on the portion of the bill above the deductible. Co-insurance for inpatient bills range from 20 percent to 10 percent as the bill increases. MediShield then pays between 80 and 90 percent of the claimable amount that exceeds the deductible.[22]

Deductibles do not apply to outpatient treatments. Instead, a 20 percent co-insurance is imposed. Only certain outpatient treatment charges are claimable under MediShield, including, for example, chemotherapy for cancer, kidney dialysis, erythropoietin for chronic kidney failure; instead, a 20 percent co-insurance is imposed.

Co-insurance, in the view of some, may impose costs that are too heavy to bear for many families (see Table 3.6 and Figures 3.1 and 3.1a).

In 2010, the average bill for hospitalization in wards Class B2 and C was about S$1,768 after subsidies. It is expected that by ages 56 to 60, most Singaporeans will have sufficient funds in their Medisave accounts to cover up to ten such hospitalizations. MediShield can be used to pay the rest. In 2010, seven out of ten bills could be paid for with MediShield and/or

Table 3.5

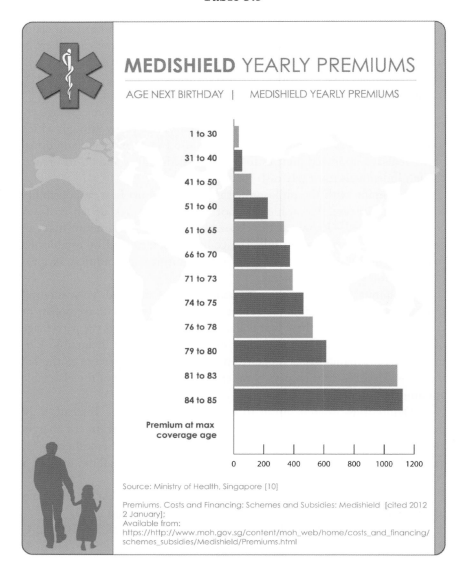

MEDISHIELD YEARLY PREMIUMS

AGE NEXT BIRTHDAY | MEDISHIELD YEARLY PREMIUMS

Source: Ministry of Health, Singapore [10]

Premiums. Costs and Financing: Schemes and Subsidies: Medishield [cited 2012 2 January];
Available from:
https://http://www.moh.gov.sg/content/moh_web/home/costs_and_financing/schemes_subsidies/Medishield/Premiums.html

Table 3.6

DEDUCTIBLE AND CO-INSURANCE

WARD CLASS

	Class C	Class B2 and Above
Deductible per policy year (aged 80 and below next birthday)	S$ 1,000	S$ 1,500
Deductible per policy year (aged 81 to 85 next birthday)	S$ 2,000	S$ 3,000
Co-Insurance Claimable anount	S$ 1,001- S$ 3,000: 20% S$ 3,001- S$ 5,000: 15% Above S$ 5,000: 10%	S$ 1,501- S$ 3,000: 20% S$ 3,001- S$ 5,000: 15% Above S$ 5,000: 10%

Source: Ministry of Health, Singapore [3]

How MediShield Works. Costs and Financing: Schemes and Subsidies: MediShield [cited 2012 2 January];

Available from:
https://http://www.moh.gov.sg/content/moh_web/home/costs_and_financing/schemes_subsidies/Medishield/How_MediShield_Works.html

Figure 3.1

HOW MEDISHIELD IS UTILIZED TO PAY FOR ONE'S HEALTHCARE BILL

CASE 1

Scenario A:
Suppose a patient is admitted to Class C ward and the total bill comes up to S$8,000 for a hospitalization in November 2009. Assuming all the expenses in the bill are within the MediShield claimable limit then the complete amount of S$8,000 can be claimed.

In this case let the policy year begin from 1 July 2009 and end on 30 June 2010.

The deductible paid by the patient in this case is S$ 1,000 since the patient is staying in Class C ward. The co-insurance payable for the total bill is calculated as:

20% of the claimable amount from S$ 1,001 to S$ 3,000
20% × S$ 2,000 = $ 400

15% of the claimable amount from S$ 3,001 to S$ 5,000
15% × S$ 2,000 = $ 300

10% of the claimable amount above $ 5,000
10% × S$ 3,000 = $ 300

Therefore, the total co-insurance payable is $1,000 (i.e. $400+$300+$300).
Thus, in this case when the total bill incurred was S$ 8,000, the patient pays S$2,000 ($1,000 as deductible and $1,000 as co-insurance).
This amount of S$2,000 can be paid either by Medisave or by cash by the patient. MediShield pays the remaining amount of S$6,000 i.e. MediShield in this case paid about 75% of the bill incurred.

Scenario B:
In Scenario A had the patient been admitted to ward B2 then the deductible would have been S$1,500. Thus, out of a total bill of $8,000 the patient would have paid S$ 2,500 and MediShield would have paid the remaining S$ 5,500.

Case 1 and 2: How MediShield is utilized to pay for one's healthcare bill [3] [1]:
General Information on MediShield Scheme. [cited 2012 2 January];
Available from:
http://ask-us.cpf.gov.sg/Home/Hybrid/themes/CPF/Uploads/Healthcare/General Information on MSH.pdf.
How MediShield Works. Costs and Financing: Schemes and Subsidies:
MediShield [cited 2012 2 January];
Available from:
https://http://www.moh.gov.sg/content/moh_web/home/costs_and_financing/schemes_subsidies/Medishield/How_MediShield_Works.html

Figure 3.1a

HOW MEDISHIELD IS UTILIZED TO PAY FOR ONE'S HEALTHCARE BILL

CASE 2

A 55-year old insured member's policy year begins from 1 July 2010 and ends on 30 June 2011. On renewal, the next policy year begins from 1 July 2011 and ends on 30 June 2012. The individual is hospitalized twice, both times in ward class B2.

Scenario A:

Both the hospitalization episodes occur in the same policy year, one in September 2010 and another in December 2010.

(i) If the Claimable amount for the first hospitalization is S$1,500 and the second one is S$2,000, the Deductible payable by the insured member for the two claims would be:

	1st Hospitalization (September 2010)	2nd Hospitalization (December 2010)
Deductable	$1,500	$0*

* The insured member has paid the full Deductible of $1,500 for the policy year. Hence, there is no Deductible payable for the second claim, which is in the same policy year.

(ii) If the claimable limit for the first hospitalization is $1,000 and the second is $2,000, the Deductible payable by the insured member for the two claims would be:

	1st Hospitalization (September 2010)	2nd Hospitalization (December 2010)
Deductable	$1,000	$500*

* The insured member has paid only part of the Deductible of $1,500 for his first claim. Hence, he has to pay the balance of $500 for his second claim, which is in the same policy year.

Scenario B:

	1st Hospitalization (September 2010)	2nd Hospitalization (August 2011)
Deductable	$1,500	$1,500*

* The insured member needs to pay the Deductible of $1,500 for the second hospitalization as it occurs in a different policy year.

Medisave without the need for the patients to pay any out-of-pocket cash for their inpatient hospitalization.[23] 90 percent of all bills were partially paid by Medisave and MediSheild in 2011.[24]

When More Coverage is Needed

MediShield can be counted on to pay off about 80 to 90 percent of claimable amounts in the subsidized Class B2/C wards. But for bills incurred in higher ward classes, individuals are encouraged to purchase Medisave-approved private insurance plans called the Integrated Shield Plans on top of MediShield. Integrated Shield Plans are enhanced, government-regulated plans that are closely linked and integrated with MediShield coverage. Five private insurers offer over 20 enhanced plans.[25] Individuals can use their Medisave dollars to purchase one (and only one) enhanced plan from among these private insurers. Claims are filed directly with the private insurer. A buyer can switch enhanced plans subject to approval by the new insurer.

Private Health Insurance

Singaporeans also have the option of purchasing purely private insurance from a number of companies. Employers in both the private and public sector generally provide this type of insurance to employees as a benefit. Even with this coverage, individuals may still enroll in MediShield and Medisave-approved Integrated Plans. One typical employer-sponsored plan is i-MediCare available from a Singapore cooperative insurance society. It is a comprehensive group medical plan covering visits to general practitioners, accident and emergency care, specialists, and hospitalization.[26]

ElderShield

Begun in 2002, ElderShield is a long-term disability insurance scheme and the government's response to the growing numbers of elderly in the population who may need help to pay for disability care. The scheme provides monthly payouts for care of people who are no longer able to perform certain daily tasks such as washing, feeding, or dressing themselves.[27] Singaporeans and permanent residents who are CPF members are automatically enrolled into the scheme when they turn 40 years old. Anyone not wishing to participate can choose to opt out.

Three private insurers run the scheme, and participants are randomly assigned to one of the insurers upon enrollment. Premiums for ElderShield are payable by Medisave dollars or cash. The premiums are affordable, are determined by the individual's age upon enrollment, and do not increase as enrollees age. Premiums are to be paid annually until age 65. Members are entitled to the benefits within the plan at any age once they have paid the requisite premiums (see Table 3.7).[28]

Covered individuals receive S$400 per month for a maximum of 72 months to pay for services such as special equipment, home nursing services, day rehabilitation, nursing homes, and more.

I have mentioned that the government is constantly looking for ways to improve the system and respond to the needs of the populace. ElderShield is an example of that kind of positive tweaking. Originally the payout was S$300 per month for a maximum of 60 months, but seeing that people needed more help, the payout was increased in 2007 to S$400 for a maximum of 72 months.

There is some question whether the new payout is enough. In the run up to the 2011 elections, there was concern expressed by an opposition party that the S$400 per month payment is too low. Some academics and industry experts have also expressed concern. The government plans to review the issue in 2013.[29]

ElderShield Supplements

In 2007, the Ministry of Health also allowed the ElderShield insurers to introduce ElderShield Supplements which gave individuals who wanted higher payouts to pay for severe-disability care the option to purchase additional coverage over and above that already provided by ElderShield. The coverage is offered through the same three private ElderShield insurers, and policies can be customized. For example, one insurer offers choices of monthly payouts from S$600 to S$3,500 (inclusive of ElderShield benefit), and a monthly payout duration fixed at 12 years or unlimited lifetime.[30]

As with the main ElderShield program, the supplements can be paid via Medisave though subject to a cap of S$600 per year per person insured, or with cash.

Medifund—The Safety Net

The third M of the Singapore healthcare systems' "3Ms" is Medifund, an endowment fund established by the government in 1993 to help individuals who cannot afford to pay for care in the most highly-subsidized wards of public hospitals. It is the system's safety net, allowing even the poorest

Table 3.7

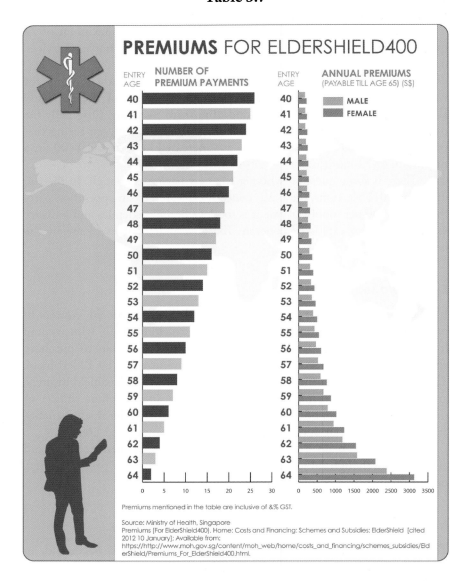

Singaporeans to receive a level of care that would otherwise be out of their reach. The program was initially funded with a S$200 million contribution by the government and now stands at about S$2 billion. Only the income generated from the Fund's principle is used for payouts.[31] The government continues its interest in helping Singapore's poorest and contributes additional dollars to Medifund from time to time. Contributions are at its discretion when budget surpluses are available. But it has recently announced the goal increasing the endowment to S$3 billion.[32] Medifund is the last resort for Singaporeans (only citizens are eligible) who are unable to pay for their subsidized healthcare bills even after using their Medisave money and their MediShield coverage. Elderly patients who have very low or no balances in their Medisave account are given priority for Medifund payouts.[33] Subsidized patients who are unable to pay for outpatient and long-term care at approved institutions can also benefit from Medifund.

Medifund Silver

Recognizing the growing numbers of the elderly in Singapore, the government has specifically set aside an amount of money in Medifund targeting assistance to individuals aged 65 and older. Named Medifund Silver, it was launched in 2007 with an initial amount of S$500 million.[34]

How Medifund Works

The eligibility criteria for patients to qualify for Medifund assistance are: the patient should be a Singapore citizen; the patient is receiving subsidized treatment; the medical treatment is received in a Medifund-approved institution, which includes intermediate and long-term care facilities, hospitals and National Specialty Centres; the patient and the family are unable to make payments for the medical bills incurred in spite of making use of the government subsidies, MediShield, and Medisave.

The Ministry of Health disburses money to the Medifund-approved institutions each year, and the Medifund Committee at each institution evaluates and approves Medifund assistance to patients.

Patients can approach the Medical Social Workers at approved institutions to receive help in navigating the application process for financial assistance. The institutions' Medifund committees screen and approve or reject applications. The amount of aid dispensed to the patient depends on the patient's and the family's income, the social circumstances of the patient, the medical condition, and the healthcare expenses incurred. The members of the Committee are independent volunteers who are active in community social work—a good idea, as such individuals are probably more familiar with the patients' situations and better able to make informed decisions. The autonomy of the Medifund Committee allows flexibility in decision-making but they must comply with the broad guidelines and directives set by the Ministry of Health.

Medifund Usage

In FY2010, some 480,000 Medifund and Medifund Silver applications were approved by the Medifund committees. The vast majority of the applications were for outpatient treatment in hospitals and institutions. Over 90 percent of the approved applications received "full help," meaning Medifund and Medifund Silver paid for 100 percent of the outstanding subsidized bills which the patient could not afford after exhausting all other means of payment. In 2009, almost S$65 million were dispersed to patients out of the S$75 million granted to healthcare institutions for their use. For inpatient treatments, the average assistance provided per application was just over S$1,000, and for outpatient treatments the average assistance per application was around S$90.

For patients facing serious cashflow problems, public hospitals may provide alternative arrangements, including installment payments, for example. This safety net is one reason why there is no documented case in Singapore of a patient being forced into bankruptcy due to the inability to pay for his healthcare bills.[35]

* * *

Chapter 3: KEY POINTS

- Medisave is a mandatory medical savings account for employed Singaporeans
  - Employees and their employers contribute a specified percentage of wages to individuals' accounts
  - Accumulated savings may be used to pay for healthcare expenses under established guidelines
  - Hospital stays, specified outpatient treatments, chronic illness treatments, various diagnostic procedures are eligible
  - Immediate family members may share and use the funds in each other's Medisave accounts

- o   The government from time to time provides "top-ups," contributing to accounts when it is able
- o   Helps patients pay for their care and at the same time keeps the whole system affordable by preventing overuse and waste

- MediShield is a voluntary, opt-out insurance program that protects patients in the case of catastrophic illness
  - o   Designed to protect patients in the most highly-subsidized hospital wards
  - o   Premiums are low and there is a lifetime cap on benefits
  - o   Deductibles, co-insurance, and claimable limits apply
  - o   Additional insurance is available through private insurers
  - o   ElderShield is a private insurance program tightly regulated by the government and offers protection against the costs of long-term disability care

- Medifund is the system's safety net
  - o   A multi-billion dollar endowment fund created by the government and designed to help the needy with their healthcare bills
  - o   Money from the Fund is provided to approved hospitals, nursing homes, and other healthcare facilities which disperse funds to indigent patients according to a strict set of guidelines and priorities

CHAPTER 4

Controlling Costs

Once a healthcare system is built, it is much more difficult to reduce fixed costs, and when those costs spiral out of control, national budgets are strained. When nations can no longer support the system they have produced, they may need to resort to unwelcome alternatives that can include long delays for appointments, testing, and treatment; rationing; limitations of service; and even denial of service.

Singapore has mostly avoided these problems. It has had the advantage of being able to build its system almost from the start, and of having a far-thinking government that carefully planned for healthcare, implemented its plans and now continually monitors, reassesses, and adjusts as necessary. The results have been outstanding. Singapore is well-known for spending a relatively small percentage of GDP on healthcare while still achieving world-class health outcomes. The total healthcare expenditure as a percentage of GDP has stayed between three and four percent since 1995. As a point of comparison, total expenditure in the United States is almost 18 percent of GDP and rising.[1]

Most of the Singapore government's spending comprises the subsidies allocated to the hospitals and polyclinics, spending on construction of healthcare facilities, and human resources. Its rigorous cost controls, as I discuss in this chapter, range from wide-scale management of the market, to regulations on how new technology is introduced to the public hospitals.

Regulating the Healthcare Marketplace

Singapore is focused on managing both public and private outlays for healthcare while at the same time keeping quality at the highest levels. The government's most consequential approach to keeping prices under control:

they have developed a quasi free market within which the healthcare system must function. The result has been better efficiency and improved delivery of care. Bureaucratic processes and structures have been replaced by a new form of healthcare marketplace.[2]

Public and private hospitals coexist in this market, but most hospital care is intentionally directed toward the public side through the patient incentives and subsidies I have described. With the ability to set the prices of services at the public hospitals, and with the ability to regulate the number of public hospitals and beds they provide, the government shapes the marketplace. It then allows market forces within that marketplace to regulate the private sector, which must not price itself out of the market. The system works because the extraordinarily high quality of the public hospitals has long been established and is scrupulously maintained.

One study comparing healthcare systems among the developed Asian nations described the Singapore government as "micro-managing provision," ensuring that public hospital charges are kept at acceptable levels, and in turn relieving pressure on Medisave accounts. It went on to say that the government "uses funding (and hospital ownership) in a calculated manner to control service costs and subsidize care, in turn limiting expenditure from insurance accounts and providing incentives for private providers to keep costs down."[3]

The effectiveness of Singapore's "micro-managing" can also be seen in the average cost of basic medical insurance—especially when compared to other countries. A study by Deutsche Bank's Global Markets Research Team and reported in *Business Insider* shows that the average annual premium for basic health insurance in Singapore is just under S$88, a cost that is just two percent of what Americans pay for their insurance.[4] See Table 4.1 for more details.

In another effort to keep the system in balance, the government has gone as far as allowing Singaporeans—starting in 2010—to use their Medisave dollars for care in overseas hospitals (owned by Singapore healthcare groups) with tie-ups with Singapore-based healthcare groups, where costs are much lower. This freedom allows Singaporeans the opportunity to benefit from lower prices and also provides a check on the costs in hospitals in Singapore itself. In order to take advantage of this opportunity, Singaporeans must first be referred by the healthcare groups' referral centers in Singapore.[5] According to the Ministry of Health, some 127 Singaporean residents used their Medisave for elective hospitalization and day surgeries in Malaysia.

Former Health Minister Khaw Boon Wan has said that the public sector should always play the dominant role in providing care services, but

Table 4.1

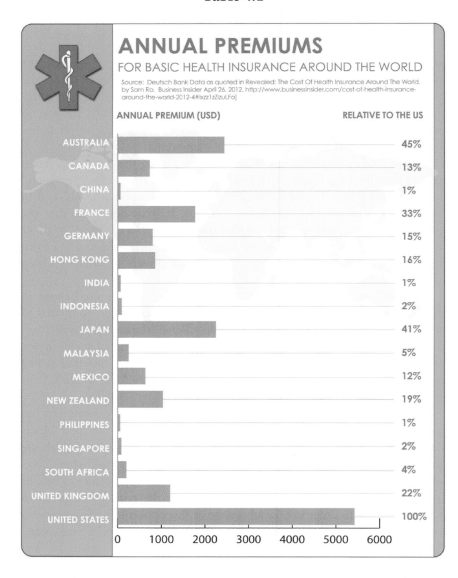

ANNUAL PREMIUMS

FOR BASIC HEALTH INSURANCE AROUND THE WORLD

Source: Deutsch Bank Data as quoted in Revealed: The Cost Of Health Insurance Around The World, by Sam Ro. Business Insider April 26, 2012. http://www.businessinsider.com/cost-of-health-insurance-around-the-world-2012-4#ixzz1zZizuLFo]

ANNUAL PREMIUM (USD)		RELATIVE TO THE US
AUSTRALIA		45%
CANADA		13%
CHINA		1%
FRANCE		33%
GERMANY		15%
HONG KONG		16%
INDIA		1%
INDONESIA		2%
JAPAN		41%
MALAYSIA		5%
MEXICO		12%
NEW ZEALAND		19%
PHILIPPINES		1%
SINGAPORE		2%
SOUTH AFRICA		4%
UNITED KINGDOM		22%
UNITED STATES		100%

there needs to be a private healthcare system to challenge it. In his view, the public sector is necessary to set the ethos for the entire system—which should not only be about maximization of profits, a primary focus of the private sector. It is the public side that tends to set boundaries and standards for ethics within the system.

Khaw takes the view that where the private sector does dominate, it will inevitably influence the government and public policy to serve its own interests. If the public healthcare system is too small, it becomes the "tail that tries to wag the dog." Once a private healthcare system becomes the dominant entrenched player, it is very difficult to unwind it—there are many vested interests and many pockets will be hurt.[6]

A dominant private sector inevitably forces higher costs and higher expenditures on the part of the government and patients, and Singapore has done an effective job of avoiding this problem.

Early Failures of the Free Market

Achieving the public–private balance that now works so successfully in Singapore took time and some major adjustments over the years. From the mid-1980s, the government "restructured" the public part of the system, giving autonomy to the hospitals for making management decisions, recruitment decisions, fixing staff remuneration, and more. The belief was that a measure of autonomy would allow public hospitals to compete effectively against one another and, in keeping with classic free market philosophy, keep costs down and the quality of services high in order to attract patients.

This freedom did lead to more competition, but it also had unexpected results: an *increase* rather than a decrease in healthcare costs. It turned out that, in their efforts to attract patients, hospitals resorted to buying expensive technology, offering new and expensive services, recruiting prominent physicians, decreasing the number of subsidized ward classes (where the less affluent went for care), and focusing attention on unsubsidized "A class" wards (that appealed to the well-off)—where they could make more profit! The "free market," it was found, did not function the way it was supposed to when it came to healthcare.[7]

The private hospitals' profit-making approach to care and rising healthcare costs were addressed in the Affordable Healthcare White Paper of 1993, which called for greater, direct government intervention in the marketplace. In the rest of this chapter, I will examine the efforts by the government to administer the quasi free market in healthcare and the other tools it uses to keep costs within reasonable bounds.

Financial Controls on Public Hospitals

In order to ensure that the hospitals do not neglect the subsidized wards in favor of the more lucrative ones, the government fixes the proportions of the different ward classes for the hospitals. It also sets guidelines for care in each ward.

The government sets subsidy and cost-recovery targets for each ward class, which indirectly keep them from producing "excess profits" associated with induced demand. The government also has policies on the use of budget surpluses. In general, the surpluses are to be used in the areas of teaching, research, and asset replacement. This ensures that "profits" are ploughed back into the healthcare system for the benefit of patients.[8]

In addition, hospitals are given annual budgets for patient subsidies, so they know how much they will be reimbursed for their expenditures on patient care. And they are required to break even within this budget.

In order for hospitals to be able to acquire expensive technology or new specialties, the government makes it necessary to seek its approval. Hospitals can apply for additional one-time grants for special equipment. Before this reform was put into place, the hospitals, according to Professor William Hsiao of Harvard's School of Public Health, competed "by offering the latest technology and expensive equipment, which appeared to be demanded by physicians and accepted by the public as an indicator of quality .... Once the new technology was put to use, it produced a higher cost inflation rate in medical services."[9]

Controlling the Availability of Doctors

The government regulates the number of medical students educated at the medical schools in the universities, and the number of foreign medical schools' degrees recognized in Singapore, all serving to control the supply of physicians in the country. The idea is that with more doctors that are available, the more likely this will "induce" demand from patients, who are less able to assess their own demand for healthcare arising from their condition compared to the medical professional. A list of medical schools recognized by the Singapore Medical Council, a statutory board under the Ministry of Health, is available at http://www.doctors.com.sg/medicalschools.html.

Doctors' Salaries

In a conversation with Mr. Anthony Tan, then Director of the Healthcare Finance and Corporate Services of the Ministry of Health, he said that the wages of doctors are reasonable and not sky-high. Doctors, however, are well-paid and rank among the top salary levels for professionals in Singapore. Specialized surgeons are amongst the highest paid people in the country, according to data from the Ministry of Manpower, which provides information on the wages of general physicians, general surgeons, specialized surgeons, and many other professionals for 2007 and 2008. It should be noted, however, that this conclusion was based on a very small sample of specialists in the private sector only. General surgeons are the third highest paid. General physicians are much lower on the list, at number 44.

General physicians earned a median monthly gross wage of S$5,000. Monthly gross wage includes basic wage, overtime payments, commissions, allowances, and other payments. The figure excludes, according to Dr. Gerald Tan who analyzed this data and blogs on the Singapore healthcare system, employers' CPF contributions, bonuses, stock options, other lump sum payments and payments-in-kind. General surgeons earned just under S$14,000 monthly. Specialized surgeons earned a median monthly gross wage of over S$22,000.[10]

Out of 100 jobs across many industries examined by the Ministry of Manpower, specialized surgeons topped the list with the highest median monthly gross wage. Managing directors came in next, with just over S$15,000. Again, it should be noted that a very small number of specialized surgeons were surveyed in 2008, in fact, only 29, compared to over 1,000 managing directors. In the survey, general surgeons were third, with just under S$14,000 monthly. For comparison purposes, a dentist's wage was S$4,500 monthly, a pharmacist S$4,100 monthly, a nurse approximately S$3,000.

The Ministry reviewed public sector physician pay in 2012, with a view to make pay in the public system more competitive with the private sector, and with a view to reward different kinds of excellence within the system: whether in clinical care, education, research, or administration.

Malpractice Costs

Malpractice can be a major cost incurred by physicians. This is especially true for doctors in the United States. Not only is malpractice very expensive, but it is also causes doctors to practice defensive medicine, often ordering many more procedures than are necessary. In Singapore, as of now, malpractice does not appear to be as costly as in the United States.

In Singapore, claims of medical malpractice are handled through the tort system. In this system, patients must sue their doctors in court and negligence must be proven in the court.[11] Negligence is one of the most common forms of malpractice in the medical professions, constituting failure to diagnose or treat a patient's illness or injury with "due care."[12] In Singapore, the approach in law to claims of medical malpractice is similar to that of the United Kingdom, Australia and the United States. The "Bolam test," developed under English law, is used to determine whether medical professionals have discharged their "duty of care"—that is, that they have performed their duties with the standard of care expected of such professionals in their treatment of a patient, and that they have used accepted practices of their profession in that treatment. Patients suing their doctors must prove that the duty of care has been breached and must also prove that the breach has caused them injury.[13]

It is up to the courts to decide whether or not a doctor has been negligent, but some observers believe that the importance the courts place on the opinions of other doctors as to whether or not negligence has taken place makes it difficult for patients to succeed in their lawsuits.[14] The malpractice policies of Singapore seem to protect both the patient and the doctor and have kept costs much lower than in many other countries. Doctors in Singapore are required to have medical malpractice insurance, but, in spite of increases over the years, the policies are still not as expensive as those in the United States.[15]

The Medical Protection Society of Singapore is the leading indemnifier of care professionals in Singapore. It is a not for profit mutual society rather than an insurance company and provides indemnity, advice, and legal representation to its members in a wide variety of situations from attacks on their reputation, to medical malpractice claims, to cases of libel.[16] Annual subscription rates vary according to the risk involved in a doctor's particular practice. For example, at the high end, a doctor in a cosmetic practice pays an annual subscription of S$32,000; a doctor with an obstetrics practice pays S$29,000; a neurosurgeon pays S$24,000; surgeons in a general practice or cardiothoracic surgery, colorectal surgery, and the like, pay just over S$7,000 annually. General practitioners pay far less: a doctor in family medicine practice pays S$1,600 each year.[17] A study by Professor Y.C. Chee provides some provocative insight into the malpractice issue. If we look at the hazards of healthcare through total lives lost per year, the risk is just over 1 in 1,000—the same, as Professor Chee notes, as bungee jumping and mountain climbing. Yet premiums for malpractice coverage from the Medical Protection Society keep rising. Here I quote from Chee's paper:

> I was comparing our MPS subscription rates for the years 2000 and 2005. The rates have risen thus. Cosmetic practice from $5,250 to $22,875. Obstetric practice from $5,250 to $20,250. Super high risk Neurosurgery from $4,500 to $16,350. Very high risk Orthopaedic and trauma surgery from $4,500 to $15,750. High risk practice from

$1,650 to $4,945. Medium risk practice from $1,200 to $2,925, Low risk practice from $700 to $1,560, and General Practice from $700 to $1,400–$1,740.[18]

The increases of two to four times over the five years from 2000 to 2005 led Dr. Chee to conclude:

> I read these increases as increase in payouts and settlements by the respective specialty practitioners to patients who have been harmed and were willing and able to seek redress through the legal system.[19]

As you can see when comparing the current subscription costs to those of previous years, costs are continuing their steep upward trend, most notably in the higher risk practices. Just to pull out two examples: obstetric practice subscriptions have gone from just over S$5,000 in 2000 to just over S$20,000 in 2005, to S$29,000 currently. Subscriptions for doctors in neurosurgery practice have increased from S$4,500 to over S$16,000 to S$24,000 today.

These numbers suggest that malpractice costs are an area of future concern. Costs are certainly rising, perhaps in reaction to social and ethical change in the country.

Transparency

The Ministry of Health publishes hospital bills on its website for medical conditions, procedures, and ward classes, including details such as charges for wards, treatment, surgery, laboratory tests and more. The average cost for the top 70 medical conditions are available (see Tables 4.2 and 4.3).

Diseases for which fewer than 30 patients were seen are not included. The information available for public hospitals is complete with all charges including doctor consultation fee. The same may not be true for the private hospitals bills, as their data is submitted on a voluntary basis.

The Ministry began publishing hospital costs in order to bring transparency into the system, empowering patients with accurate information for making informed decisions regarding good-quality, low-cost treatment. The published information also encourages competition between healthcare institutions, motivating them to bring down the costs. These cost comparisons might be used in other advanced economies as a point of reference.

Hospital Ward Choices

I discussed in Chapter 3 that the public hospitals of Singapore offer a range of room accommodations (from private to dormitory-style rooms), with

Table 4.2

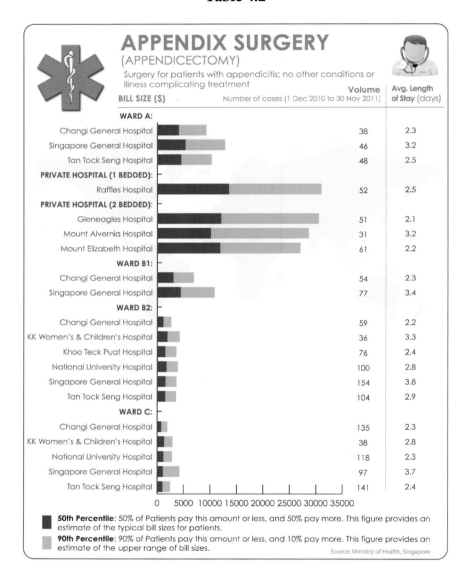

APPENDIX SURGERY
(APPENDICECTOMY)

Surgery for patients with appendicitis; no other conditions or illness complicating treatment

BILL SIZE ($)	Volume Number of cases (1 Dec 2010 to 30 Nov 2011)	Avg. Length of Stay (days)
WARD A:		
Changi General Hospital	38	2.3
Singapore General Hospital	46	3.2
Tan Tock Seng Hospital	48	2.5
PRIVATE HOSPITAL (1 BEDDED):		
Raffles Hospital	52	2.5
PRIVATE HOSPITAL (2 BEDDED):		
Gleneagles Hospital	51	2.1
Mount Alvernia Hospital	31	3.2
Mount Elizabeth Hospital	61	2.2
WARD B1:		
Changi General Hospital	54	2.3
Singapore General Hospital	77	3.4
WARD B2:		
Changi General Hospital	59	2.2
KK Women's & Children's Hospital	36	3.3
Khoo Teck Puat Hospital	76	2.4
National University Hospital	100	2.8
Singapore General Hospital	154	3.8
Tan Tock Seng Hospital	104	2.9
WARD C:		
Changi General Hospital	135	2.3
KK Women's & Children's Hospital	38	2.8
National University Hospital	118	2.3
Singapore General Hospital	97	3.7
Tan Tock Seng Hospital	141	2.4

0   5000 10000 15000 20000 25000 30000 35000

50th Percentile: 50% of Patients pay this amount or less, and 50% pay more. This figure provides an estimate of the typical bill sizes for patients.

90th Percentile: 90% of Patients pay this amount or less, and 10% pay more. This figure provides an estimate of the upper range of bill sizes.

Source: Ministry of Health, Singapore

Table 4.3

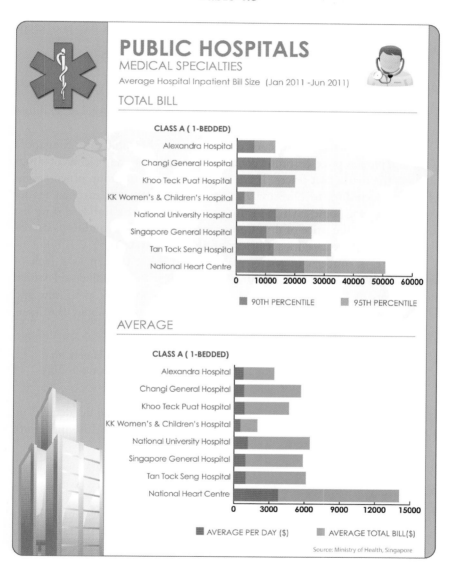

PUBLIC HOSPITALS
MEDICAL SPECIALTIES
Average Hospital Inpatient Bill Size (Jan 2011 -Jun 2011)

TOTAL BILL

CLASS A (1-BEDDED)

Alexandra Hospital
Changi General Hospital
Khoo Teck Puat Hospital
KK Women's & Children's Hospital
National University Hospital
Singapore General Hospital
Tan Tock Seng Hospital
National Heart Centre

0   10000   20000   30000   40000   50000   60000

■ 90TH PERCENTILE   ■ 95TH PERCENTILE

AVERAGE

CLASS A (1-BEDDED)

Alexandra Hospital
Changi General Hospital
Khoo Teck Puat Hospital
KK Women's & Children's Hospital
National University Hospital
Singapore General Hospital
Tan Tock Seng Hospital
National Heart Centre

0   3000   6000   9000   12000   15000

■ AVERAGE PER DAY ($)   ■ AVERAGE TOTAL BILL($)

Source: Ministry of Health, Singapore

a range of amenities and corresponding prices, but with the same quality of care. This allows consumers to consider value in their choices. Financial counselors, who are trained frontline admissions staff at the hospitals, provide patients with estimates of the costs they will most likely incur in the course of their stay, and the patients can decide which wards are within their means. The ability to choose aligns costs with patients' ability to pay and keeps unnecessary expenditures in check.

Prescription Drugs

Prescription drugs represent about 18 percent of Singapore's total expenditure on healthcare.

Unlike in its effort to control the costs of hospital care, Singapore does not pursue price or profit control measures over the pricing of drugs and lets the market set prices. There is, however, a lot of group procurement of drugs, according to Director Tan in our interview, via an open tender system, allowing some savings in this area. Drugs on the standard drug list are subsidized. The price of drugs prescribed for common conditions can be found on the Pharmaceutical Society of Singapore website.[20]

There is concern in some quarters over what is seen as a lack of transparency in decisions regarding which drugs to subsidize and which not. Society at large, it is argued, is being kept in the dark as to how and why decisions are made. Dr. Jeremy Lin recently wrote about the issue, noting that

> In Singapore, bureaucrats determine subsidy decisions in a largely top-down, opaque fashion, adopting a 'Trust us, we know best' approach. This is in stark contrast to the approach taken by other countries.

He argues that Singaporeans "collectively as a society should decide" on the values governing such decisions that may well have life-and-death consequences.[21]

Mandatory Insurance

In another cost control measure, it became mandatory in 2008 for employers to purchase medical insurance for low-income foreign workers, such as construction workers and maids. The regulation covers all new foreign workers as well as those already in Singapore, numbering approximately 650,000 at the time. As this regulation was going into effect, the government was ending subsidies for foreign workers in the public hospitals and polyclinics. The insurance ensures that the burden of caring for foreigners who cannot afford care is not carried by the citizens or the government.

The regulation initially stipulated that coverage of at least S$5,000 per year be provided but was increased to S$15,000 in 2010. The insurance covers inpatient care and day surgery. Statistics showed that foreign workers were hospitalized most often for dengue fever, appendicitis, and stomach flu.[22]

The government worked with private insurance companies to ensure that affordable policies would be available for purchase, and employers are able to choose from a variety of policies as long as government minimums (S$15,000 of coverage for inpatient care and day surgery) are met. The regulation is administered by the Ministry of Manpower.

Cost-Saving Technologies

Singapore continually pursues cost-saving technologies for the healthcare system, including information technology initiatives such as a national electronic-health-record system. It establishes a continuum of care, meeting the goal of "one patient one record."

Investing in an Electronic System for Patient Records

There is no more current topic in healthcare today than the development of electronic health records. Here again, Singapore is a leader, investing heavily in a technology platform that will realize the goal of "one patient, one record," enabling care integration and enabling a continuum of care for every patient. Patients' health records are stored on a nationwide electronic medical record system.

According to Dr. Sarah Muttitt, then Chief Information Officer at the Information Systems Division, MOH Holdings, Singapore's National Electronic Health Record program is "clinically led and internationally connected." She told me that in her view, the system must be all about quality and safety and security of information. Her mission is to build the "backbone" of the system, allowing for the input and exchange of information from many sources, and providing users an integrated view of the information. Her division, she said, has a ten-year masterplan to develop the system and provide functionality throughout the healthcare system. She estimated the cost at S$400 per patient, a reasonable sum of money. According to a Ministry statement, the government will fund the bulk of the capital costs of the new system directly, with the healthcare providers funding the balance.

In the sixth year, she believed they will see a return on investment as they will begin to see cost savings through medication management, compliance and innovations in the home, made possible by the electronic health record system. A patient's personal health record needs to be accessible and provide health services through the nearest GP. Dr. Muttitt told me that that looking ahead, "one part of Electronic Health Record program is what we call, 'one citizen one inbox,' where you can perform many parallel activities involving taxes, land authorities, licensing things. We try to aggregate."[23]

The system keeps records of all the medical conditions including the latest list of medications being taken for chronic diseases treatment. The records are updated every time the patients have medical tests or see a doctor. The record is stored in a format that is accessible and can be updated by any registered public or private medical institution in Singapore, when fully rolled out. Patients will also be able to access their own electronic records from home via a computer or mobile phone. Patients will be able to see their medical history, screening results, prescription test and measures for pre-emptive intervention, for example medication instructions and other information for dealing with asthma. Patients would be able to keep weight, clinical indicators such as blood glucose levels, and Asthma Control Test scores up to date, allowing distance-monitoring by care professionals.

Investing in TeleMedicine

In 2008, the Ministry of Health established Integrated Health Information Systems (IHIS) to oversee the development of healthcare services through technology within the public healthcare sector. Numerous pilot programs are now in place throughout the Singapore healthcare system using computers, electronic transmissions, videoconferencing equipment, and tablet computers for long-distance doctor–patient interactions as well as doctor–specialist interactions and consultations.

Most polyclinics in Singapore are already transmitting x-ray images via computer to radiology centers to be interpreted, but this is just the tip of the iceberg.

Several pilot programs now give patients the opportunity to "tele-consult" with specialists in hospitals from their home or from a nearby polyclinic. In one program aimed at the bedridden elderly, a nurse is sent to a bedridden patient's home with a tablet computer, examines the patient, and then connects with the patient's doctor to report her results on camera. In one documented case, the cost of this service was S$65, versus over S$200 for the cost of a physician's house call.

Other uses of telemedicine now taking place in Singapore include emergency doctors treating stroke patients in consultation with specialists at other locations via videoconferencing and the transmission of scans sent to the specialists.

In another program, the National Healthcare Group Eye Institute is using telemedicine and finding that certain abnormalities of the eye can be detected from images transmitted to specialists just as well as in a face-to-face consultation.[24]

Good results are also being found in dermatology examinations in a program initiated by the Institute of Mental Health, whereby patients are not required to leave their facility for an examination, usually a stressful and expensive endeavor.[25]

If proven effective, further telemedicine capabilities will be rolled out to more hospitals and other healthcare facilities, with the potential for lowering costs, speeding up diagnoses and treatments, and providing immobile patients with high-quality care.

Controlling Demand

Along with the many measures I have discussed in this chapter for controlling costs on what can be called the "supply side" of healthcare—the hospitals, doctors, polyclinics, etc.—there are numerous ways the government keeps the "demand" side in check—the behaviors of patients and potential consumers of healthcare. They have been presented in detail in Chapter 3, but it is worth listing them again in this context. They include co-payments, deductibles, and tight restrictions on the uses of Medisave and MediShield for consultations, treatments, and procedures. These controls are perhaps just as important as what I call the quasi free market in healthcare in controlling costs in that they perform the role of discouraging unnecessary doctor visits, tests, and treatments. The result is a more careful use of the system's resources by healthcare consumers.

The government has always made clear that a welfare system or an entitlement mentality has no place in Singapore. The need for "individual responsibility" and "self-reliance" on the part of the citizenry in all personal matters, including healthcare, has always been an integral factor in the country's achievements.

Insisting that patients pay their share of their healthcare costs is indicative of this philosophy and has resulted in prudent use of the system. Another result is a relatively high amount of private expenditure for care. Private expenditure, as a percentage of the total health expenditure, was about 65 percent in 2010, including payments from MediShield, Integrated Shield Plans, Medisave, other third-party payers and employer benefits, rising from about 50 percent in 1995.

Maintaining the High Quality of Care

I began this chapter saying that the healthcare market put into place by the government works because the quality of public care remains very high throughout the system. Strong regulatory bodies and regulations are in place to make sure that the high standards are maintained. Singapore, in fact, has invested itself in continual quality improvement in healthcare. According to M.K. Lim, the first National Quality Control Circle Convention took place in 1982. Every hospital and specialist center has a committee to address quality issues. The focus is not only on service quality but also on improving clinical quality. Teams of quality managers in hospitals measure clinical processes and outcomes.

Since 2000, the Ministry of Health has mandated that all private and public hospitals participate in the Maryland Quality Indicator Project which involves the monitoring of a set of clinical quality indicators and benchmarking those indicators against national and international norms. The indicators include: inpatient mortality; perioperative mortality; unscheduled return to the operating theater; unscheduled readmission within 15 days; unscheduled admission following ambulatory procedure; inpatient admission following unscheduled returns to the accident and emergency department; and device utilization and device associated infection in the intensive care unit.[26]

The Ministry has also set up a "Healthcare Quality Improvement and Innovation Fund" which invites applicants (professionals and institutions) annually to submit proposals for funding pilot innovative clinical quality improvement projects for improving the standards, quality, and safety of patient care within and across the healthcare systems and sectors.[27]

A good example of the ongoing commitment to improving quality of care has been the Singapore National Asthma Program. The program was launched in 2001 to find ways to lessen the high burden of asthma in the country, which has one of the highest rates of asthma deaths in the world. One aspect of the effort was improving individuals' control over the disease through the use of inhaled corticosteroids as a preventative against asthma attacks. As a low-cost intervention effort, the program has been deemed a success.[28]

In the case of diabetes, we can see once again the system making advances in the quality and delivery of care. Diabetes mellitus sufferers constitute over 11 percent of the 18 to 69 age group, increasing from eight percent in 2004.[29] Diabetes is the seventh leading cause of death, with over 3.5 percent of all deaths attributable to the disease.[30] In 2005, the National Healthcare Group began to build a diabetes registry with the intention of improving continuity of care and producing better measurement of outcomes. The system collects patient records, test results, key reminders for future tests and screenings for physicians' use. It also reports outcomes in a way that allows the data to be used for quality improvement and more effective management of the patient pool.[31] These efforts are admirable and exhibit the responsiveness of the system. In spite of these programs, the treatment of diabetes remains a difficult challenge, with the incidence of the disease continuing to trend upward and with Singaporeans continuing to exhibit a growing number of complications from the disease.

Concern has been expressed over disparities in economic status and immigrant status of patients possibly being reflected in disparities in care. One study looked at the time factor involved in treating myocardial infarction—heart attack—among patients of differing socioeconomic groups. No differences were found in quality of care—including pathway to hospital admission and treatment. The study also looked at the time it took from the appearance of symptoms in the patients until coronary intervention took place. Here differences were found, with longer waiting times for permanent residents versus Singapore-born residents, suggesting the need for a "tailored approach to healthcare resource allocation" among the different migrant classes in Singapore.[32]

M.K. Lim, writing in 2004, suggested that the following advances are still needed to improve quality and patient safety: "strengthening of the evidence base for quality initiatives (for example, through rigorous program evaluation); greater civil society involvement (for example, voluntary accreditation); greater patient empowerment (for example, through greater transparency with respect to publishing of hospital quality indicators)."[33]

And yet, whatever its faults may be, the system is working and working extremely well. The country's efforts to improve the health outcomes for its people can be seen in the declining rates of "amenable mortality"—that is, the death rate from causes that can be treated medically. One study examining mortality rates in the country from 1965 to 1994 found that death rates were being reduced through timely medical intervention for treatable conditions such as bronchitis, ulcer, pneumonia, asthma, appendicitis, and other conditions. In effect, Singapore is improving the health of its people through timely care.

Gains were more significant for these treatable conditions than for "preventable" areas such as lung cancer, chronic liver disease, or motor vehicle injury. But this finding was in line with trends in European countries, where amenable mortality also declined more than preventable mortality.

Two disparities that should be noted: the study found gender and ethnic differences in amenable mortality. Decline in death rates from some diseases was less in women than in men, and the Chinese showed the best results in the years of the study, over Malays and Indians.[34]

In the area of mental health, it has been suggested that the mental health system in Singapore lacks coordination and is underdeveloped in certain areas.[35] The Ministry of Health, however, in 2007, launched a National Mental Health Blueprint to improve the state of mental health services within Singapore's communities. According to former Health Minister Khaw Boon Wan, much has been improved, but there is much still to be done. In a recent speech, he stated that "We need to detect patients early, so that there is timely intervention. We need to reduce the stigma surrounding mental illness, so that the patients can be more confident to come forward for treatment and after receiving treatment, to integrate back into the community." He noted that under the Blueprint, programs are now in development and implementation in the communities to bring about early detection and to initiate treatment. Four programs have been developed that separately target and treat children, youths, adults, and the elderly.[36]

The Ministry of Health conducts an annual Patient Satisfaction Survey, in Singapore's public healthcare institutions. The survey assesses the level of patient satisfaction with the healthcare services, compares performance of the institutions, and collects suggestions for improvement. Patients' opinions are recorded on nine service quality attributes: facilities, care coordination, knowledge and skills of doctors, care and concern shown by doctors, knowledge and skills of nurses, care and concern shown by nurses, knowledge and skills of allied health professionals, clear explanation by staff on the procedures and care.[37]

In the 2010 Patient Satisfaction Survey, the highest overall patient satisfaction for a hospital was 82 percent. Overall, eight out of ten patients in public hospitals, polyclinics, and national specialty centers said that they would recommend the services at the public healthcare institutions to others.

Another study—somewhat older than the Patient Satisfaction Survey—suggests that Singaporeans are unconcerned about the share of healthcare costs they are expected to shoulder under the principle of individual responsibility. According to the study, they appear content to pay their portion of healthcare costs plus more if and when they desire higher levels of service.[38] A strong regulatory environment in Singapore also encourages a strong culture of high standards. Boards enforce professional healthcare standards, including the Singapore Nursing Board, Singapore Dental Board, and Singapore Pharmacy Board. Medical doctors and nurses, and recently allied health workers are encouraged to continually improve their skills via programs like the Health Manpower Development Program. Doctors undergo compulsory continuing medical education in order to be re-certified. The Ministry of Health publishes clinical practice guidelines to encourage the practice of evidence-based medicine.

The Health Sciences Authority is tasked with ensuring the safety of drugs and medical devices and that these health products meet the requisite standards of safety, efficacy, and quality. Products may require a full evaluation or may qualify for a shortened process if they have already been approved by certain other nations' drug regulatory agencies. Even after approval, the Authority maintains a system to track problems and issues related to the product. It also collaborates with international organizations and experts to ensure product safety. Once a product is approved, healthcare professionals in both the private and public sectors are free to prescribe it.

* * *

Chapter 4: KEY POINTS

- Singapore has developed a quasi free market for healthcare that enables it to control costs and keep quality high
    - o Public and private hospitals coexist in this market, but public dominates because of carefully crafted patient incentives and subsidies plus price controls on treatment
    - o The private sector is kept in check as it competes against public sector advantages
    - o Stringent quality controls in the public system help maintain the public/private balance

- An early attempt allowing the public hospitals to compete freely against one another led to higher costs and exclusionary tactics as hospitals focused on serving the affluent, where most profit could be made

- Financial controls on public hospitals help keep costs within acceptable bounds
    - o The government fixes the proportion of different ward classes, sets guidelines for care along with ward charges in public hospitals

- o The government determines the number of beds in public hospitals
- o Public hospitals are given annual budgets for patient subsidies
- o Approval must be sought before acquiring expensive technology or developing new medical specialties

- The number of medical students and the number of doctors licensed in Singapore are tightly regulated
- Cost transparency helps patients make choices
  - o The Ministry of Health publishes hospital bills on its website
  - o At point of consumption, hospital ward choices are clearly explained to patients along with estimated cost

- Neither price nor profit controls are pursued over prescription drugs
  - o Group procurement allows for some savings through bulk purchasing

- In order to protect the system against rising costs, employers are required to provide foreign workers with medical insurance

- Investments in technologies such as telemedicine and an Electronic System for Patient Records are showing great promise for improving the quality of care and lowering costs

- The government controls demand for healthcare through the use of co-payments, deductibles, and tight restrictions on the uses of Medisave and MediShield
  - o The controls result both in prudent use of medical resources by consumers and a high level of private healthcare expenditure vs. government/public expenditure

- Singapore invests in continual quality improvement of healthcare through numerous programs and initiatives plus very high standards for care professionals
  - o These efforts ensure that cost controls do not damage the high quality of care that has been achieved

CHAPTER 5

Financing

The Government of Singapore contributes billions of dollars to building and maintaining the country's healthcare system and subsidizing a major portion of the cost of patient care, based on the individual's ability to pay. As discussed earlier, the country does all this and achieves world-class outcomes while spending far less than most developed nations.

One of the many factors that contribute to Singapore's healthcare budgets remaining within reasonable bounds is that consumers of care are asked to pay their share for services. Private expenditure on healthcare amounts to over 65 percent of the total national expense of healthcare.

At the same time that the government asks its people to share in the expense of their care, it has also developed tools and programs for them to do so. Medisave, the mandatory medical savings program, MediShield, the opt-out catastrophic health insurance scheme, and Medifund, the government endowment fund to aid the indigent, are critical vehicles for helping the people of Singapore with their healthcare expenses.

In this chapter, I will examine the structure of funding mechanisms and subsidies that ensures the affordability of care and at the same time maintains the high-quality, state-of-the-art delivery system.

Government Subsidies

I spoke with Mr. Anthony Tan, then Director of the Healthcare Finance and Corporate Services of the Ministry of Health, and asked him about the government's approach to subsidies. He told me that "the healthcare financing philosophy aims to provide universal healthcare coverage. We have heavy subsidies for basic services in all sectors, but the individual has a responsibility."

The delicate balance between universal coverage and individual responsibility is constantly monitored and adjusted to meet changing conditions. This is done through adjustments to subsidy levels, eligibility of institutions, treatments covered, and more. Here is a rundown on the current status of the Singapore healthcare subsidy program. The government pays direct subsidies to public hospitals, polyclinics, and other healthcare providers to reimburse a portion of their costs for treating their patients. The funding structure is a hybrid system of block grants and Casemix, a method for classifying and describing the "output" of the provider. About 70 medical conditions are financed through Casemix.

According to the Ministry of Health, hybrid block grants are allocated to public hospitals: part of their annual budget is given in the form of a block, with the remainder on a piece-rate basis for 70 common conditions based on Diagnosis-Related Groups (DRG). DRG is a system used to classify inpatient and day surgery cases into one of over 600 approximate groupings according to the patients' diagnosis and treatment. Year-on-year data for all DRGs are collected, along with data on accident and emergency care and specialist outpatient clinic care. The hybrid block budgets are reviewed every three to five years based on the actual workload of the institutions. Hospitals are allowed to keep their surpluses, which they can generate, for example, from the subsidized wards by lowering their costs. In addition to the block budget, other funds are available for manpower development and research.

These subsidies become available to the public in a number of ways: for acute and inpatient care in specific ward classes in the public hospitals; for outpatient care in public hospitals and at polyclinics; emergency care at all public hospitals (subsidized at a flat rate for all patients irrespective of their immigration status); intermediate- and long-term care at facilities managed by Voluntary Welfare Organizations (on a case-by-case basis); means-tested patients at private nursing homes (under the Ministry of Health's portable subsidy program). In addition, care by private sector primary care physicians is also subsidized for Health Assist cardholders under the Community Health Assist Scheme (CHAS).

Hospitals

As presented earlier, there are five ward classes in restructured hospitals: C, B2, B2+, B1, and A. Class C wards are highly subsidized to 80 percent. The subsidy decreases gradually for the different wards (see Table 5.1), with Class A wards offering no subsidies to patients. Means testing determines eligibility and amount of subsidy for each patient.

Table 5.1

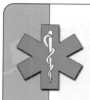

SUBSIDIES AT PUBLIC HOSPITALS

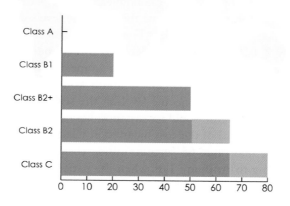

Class Ward	Subsidy Level
Class A	0%
Class B1	20%
Class B2+	50%
Class B2	65%- 50% *
Class C	80%- 65% *

* Means-tested

Source: Ministry of Health, Singapore

Means testing does not prevent patients from choosing a ward class of their choice. High-income earners, for example, can choose the C class ward, but the amount of subsidy provided would be lower, as would the amenities in the ward. Lower-income patients can choose one of the least subsidized wards, if they can pay for it. According to the Ministry of Health, if patients choose to stay in a private ward, their income is not checked. They are free to choose the private ward but they would be asked to make a deposit. The hospital admissions office or financial counselor advises the patient on the amount of the bill that can be incurred and the patient is free to choose. Patients who want to avail themselves of the maximum subsidy will have their income checked with their consent.

In order to ensure subsidies are directed to people in need, means testing was introduced in 2009. Economically active patients hospitalized in Class C and B2 wards would have their income levels checked, with their consent, through Central Provident Fund records. For self-employed patients, the subsidy is based on incomes declared for tax purposes. Non-working patients have the annual value of their home taken into consideration. Patients earning more than S$3,200 a month would begin to see the subsidy decreased. At the highest income level on the scale, patients earning more than S$5,200 per month would receive subsidies of 65 percent (instead of the maximum 80 percent) of the cost incurred in Class C wards, and 50 percent (instead of the maximum 65 percent of their costs in B2 wards.[1]

According to Anthony Tan, when the patients are retired from work, subsidies are based on their property type, or the "annual value" of their homes, as determined by the Singapore tax authorities. Annual value is defined as the estimated annual rent of a property if it were rented out, excluding the furniture, furnishings and maintenance fees.[2] Patients with homes below or equal to S$13,000 in annual value receive the maximum subsidy. Above S$13,000, they receive the minimum levels (50 percent for class B2, and 65 percent for class C).[3] The hospital admissions office or financial counselor advises the patients on the most appropriate, affordable ward class given the patients' circumstances and medical condition.

Polyclinics

Consumers visiting polyclinics (where outpatient care is provided) are eligible for subsidies for the cost of medical consultation, basic investigations, and drugs. Patients are liable for co-payments for medical consultations and drugs. Citizens over 65 and children younger than 18 are entitled to a subsidy of up to 75 percent, while the rest of the citizens receive up to

50 percent subsidy. A discussion of polyclinics and their fees and subsidies follows in Chapter 6.

Drugs

The government also provides subsidies to patients for the cost of drugs. The amount depends on patients' paying status and the programs under which the drug is covered, for example, the "Standard Drug List," or the "Medication Assistance Fund" (which helps the poor pay for expensive drugs). Covered drugs comprise up to 90 percent of the total volume of medication prescriptions.[4] Some drugs are subsidized for specific clinical indications.

Since February 2012, Health Assist cardholders have been eligible for higher subsidies at the public healthcare institutions should they need selected drugs for the management of their chronic condition covered under the CHAS scheme. Needy patients who are eligible for the Medication Assistance Fund will have drug subsidies raised to 75 percent.

The Ministry of Health maintains a Standard Drug List designed along the lines of the World Health Organization's Essential Drugs List, which enumerates cost-effective drugs considered basic therapies for the management of common diseases. The Ministry has a Drug Advisory Committee that reviews the Standard Drug List yearly, with input from pharmacological and medical organizations, and considers whether proposed drugs are essential for the treatment of medical conditions relevant to diseases and mortality in Singapore; whether the drug is superior to existing standard drugs; whether the long-term safety of the drug has been established; and the results of a cost-benefit analysis.

One side note: a study of five public-sector hospitals has found that the rate of prescription of broad-spectrum antibiotics in the hospitals is higher than that of European hospitals. This may be due to high rates of antimicrobial resistance, but more research will be necessary to understand the causes of the trend and what to do about it.[5]

Permanent Residents

Permanent residents also benefit from the government's system of subsidies, though the subsidy offered to them is lower than that offered to Singapore citizens. In its 2012 budget, the government announced a lowering of the subsidy rates for permanent residents in order to sharpen the distinction in benefits received between citizens and permanent residents. The differential is meant to convey to citizens that they will always be accorded higher priority.

These new adjustments pertain to inpatient services, that is, Class B2 and C wards, day surgery and specialist outpatient clinics in the public hospitals, as well as intermediate and long-term care services. With this adjustment, the government estimates that the subsidy for most permanent residents will be half the corresponding subsidy that citizens receive. Subsidies are the same, however, for accident and emergency care.[6]

A Look at the Healthcare Budget

As I am writing this book, the 2012 healthcare budget is in effect. The expected expenditures for the year total S$4.7 billion representing just one and one-third percent of GDP. The operating budget is just over S$4 billion, and the development budget is almost S$650 million. The previous year's budget was S$4 billion, or just under one and one-quarter percent of GDP.[7]

The Ministry spends these dollars on subsidies, promoting good health practices, education, and building up and maintaining a strong public health infrastructure. Below are highlights of the budgeted expenditures. I hope it will prove useful to readers to see how Singapore's Ministry of Health plans its spending to ensure that the healthcare system maintains its high quality and also adjusts to meet the changing needs of the populace.

Close to S$3 billion will be spent on subsidies for Singaporeans seeking medical care at polyclinics, public hospitals, and all other eligible institutions; S$600 million for a top up to the Medifund capital sum, enabling S$20 million more to be disbursed each year; just over S$200 million for programs that promote health throughout the population, through preventative measures such as vaccination programs and education.

Efforts are underway to expand healthcare facilities generally, building new ones and upgrading existing ones. The development budget is be devoted to these efforts which (at the time of writing) include major projects such as the development of the Singapore General Hospital Pathology Building, the redevelopment of the National Heart Centre, and the building of nursing homes, day care and rehabilitation facilities, and senior activity centers to better serve the growing numbers of elderly people.

Tweaking the System

A budget or spending plan is an opportunity to make adjustments in the organization being funded. This budget is an ongoing effort to adjust to the realities of the growing percentages of elderly in Singapore's population. The challenge becomes increasing the capacity and capabilities of the system to care for these people, funding the necessary expansion, and helping the families of the elderly shoulder the burden of costs of the care.

The initiatives for the elderly seem to support the notion that the system is well-managed and responsive to changing conditions in the environment. In his speech introducing the national budget, the Deputy Prime Minister acknowledged that while bed capacity in the acute hospitals would be increased, "we must also shift from the current concentration on acute hospital care and move towards providing affordable, long term care. Most importantly, we must make it easier and more affordable for the elderly to stay at home, with access to quality care services when needed."[8]

The 2012 Budget provided for higher subsidies for intermediate- and long-term care, increased and improved care infrastructure, more doctors and nurses added to the system with competitive pay, and new subsidies extended to the middle class making care more affordable than in the past.

Some specifics include: adding 1,900 beds in the public acute hospitals by 2020, a 30 percent increase; adding 1,800 beds to community hospitals, a 100 percent increase; increasing subsidies to the community hospitals; and increasing subsidies for nursing homes, home-based and community-based care, including providing S$120 per month for paying foreign domestic helpers to care for an elderly member at home. There will be subsidies for installing elderly-friendly features in the home. From 2012, regular annual Medisave top-ups of up to S$450 will also be provided to elderly Singaporeans to help with their healthcare expenses under the GST Voucher Scheme. 85 percent of all elderly Singaporeans aged above 65 will be eligible for the top up. The Minister also announced that the healthcare budget will be increased to about S$8 billion over the next five years.

Medical Tourism

Medical tourism is a growth industry for Singapore. The country has become a leading destination for foreigners seeking high-quality care at costs much lower than what they would have to pay in their home countries. Companies now market "sun and surgery" travel packages and make arrangements for medical care at hospitals in Singapore as well as India, Thailand, and other international destinations.[9]

Likewise, better-off patients from less-developed countries in the region such as Indonesia and Malaysia come to Singapore for high-quality specialist care not available in their own countries.[10]

Looking at comparative costs, it is easy to see why Asia has become an important destination for patients seeking lower cost medical treatment.

One study found that charges for common procedures such as a heart bypass might cost US$11,000 in Thailand vs. US$130,000 in the United States. A knee replacement operation can cost US$13,000 in Singapore as opposed to US$40,000 in the United States.[11]

In 2010, over 700,000 medical tourists traveled to Singapore and spent an estimated S$940 million in the country. The spending figure represents an increase of over S$200 million from 2009.[12] There is considerable potential for future growth. Consulting firm KPMG estimates that the global medical tourism industry is growing at a rate of 20 to 30 percent annually and is now a US$100 billion industry.[13]

Singapore has been forward-looking in its vision to turn itself into a regional hub for medical services, and it has encouraged the development of private sector specialized services to support the industry.[14]

Singapore's biomedical initiative has, among other advantages, resulted in advances in stem-cell research that has stalled in other countries. These efforts have led to a number of leading edge treatments, especially for cancer, that are not available elsewhere.[15]

In 2006, over 400,000 medical tourists from 60 different countries sought treatment in Singapore.[16] The top four countries sending patients are Indonesia, Malaysia, the United States/Canada, and the United Kingdom.[17] The number of medical tourists arriving from China and Middle East has been on the rise.

The private hospitals are the main players in medical tourism, but the public sector has a role as well. According to research by Nomura Asia Healthcare, about 30 percent of the patients at Singapore's private Parkway hospitals and 60 to 40 percent in Raffles Hospital are foreigners.[18]

The numbers available for the public hospitals indicate that they treated about 20 percent of all medical tourists in 2002.[19]

Aside from the obvious benefit of injecting foreign dollars into the economy, medical tourism is important for other reasons. With Singapore's small population, it would be much more difficult to support the expense of maintaining its high-quality care system without the influx of foreigners. With a larger pool of patients, economies of scale come into play, generally lowering costs and at the same time providing more services for all. The addition of foreign patients also allows doctors to sub-specialize. Also key is the fact that expensive, advanced technology becomes more cost efficient if it is allowed to serve greater numbers of patients. In effect, Singaporeans themselves benefit when they open their hospital doors to medical tourists.[20]

The success of medical tourism has caused some tensions in the country as Singaporeans see foreigners in their public hospitals and believe they are subsidizing their care. They also experience longer waits at the hospitals, day surgery clinics, and outpatient clinics and want to blame the attention now being paid to outsiders. Is medical tourism, then, affecting the quality of their care?

Government officials have had to address these concerns and reassure the public of their commitment to the citizenry with regard to healthcare services. Former Health Minister Khaw Boon Wan stated in Parliament: "we will never neglect local patients and simply chase the foreign patient load."[21] On another occasion, he told Parliament that the public hospitals were not included in overseas marketing campaigns, and that foreign patients represent less than three percent of the total public hospital patient load.[22] Singapore does not practice differential pricing for foreign patients—they are simply not eligible for subsidies.[23]

Competition

Singapore is facing increased price competition from neighboring countries: Thailand, Philippines, Malaysia, and India. Medical care for foreigners is more expensive in Singapore than in other Asian countries that have a reputation for offering excellent medical services to foreigners—Thailand and India specifically. Nonetheless, Singapore has some advantages beyond the high quality of care it provides. Singapore is known as an orderly, law-abiding society with an English-speaking environment, facts that offer reassurance and provide a level of confidence to travelers from other nations. In addition, the system's high-end amenities appeal to many medical tourists from developed countries.[24]

* * *

Chapter 5: Key Points

- Singapore's healthcare system is financed through both public and private expenditure

- The government helps individuals with the cost of their care through a system of subsidies

  - The aim of the subsidies is universal care coverage combined with individual responsibility

  - The government provides funds directly to public hospitals, polyclinics, and other providers to reimburse their costs for treating patients

- o   Subsidies (government subvention) are given through a system of block grants and Casemix funding to hospitals
- o   Casemix is a way of classifying and describing hospital "output"

- The 2012 budget is S$4.7 billion, just one and one-third percent of GDP
  - o   The operating portion of the budget is just over S$4 billion
  - o   The development budget is approximately S$650 million

- The government carefully adjusts its healthcare budgets to meet changing conditions
  - o   A current adjustment is the move toward providing high-quality long-term care for the elderly through expansion of facilities and related subsidies

- Singapore has become a leading destination for foreigners seeking medical treatment
  - o   Medical tourists seeking high-quality care have become an important source of revenue
  - o   The industry's development is being encouraged by the government

CHAPTER 6

Design and Infrastructure

Primary Healthcare

Private General Practitioners

Primary care, where ill patients make first contact with care professionals, is largely issued by private rather than public care providers. There are approximately 2,000 private general practitioners in Singapore, located mainly in housing estates, and they deliver 80 percent of primary care.[1] Several private general practitioner chains serve the public, including Raffles Medical (with more than 70 clinics), Parkway Shenton (over 40 clinics), and Frontier Healthcare Group (with nine clinics). The idea behind allowing the private sector to handle much of this care stems from the philosophy that people must take responsibility for their own health. It follows that patients should pay for minor episodic ailments on their own and not rely on government subsidies to defray the cost.

Ailments that the general practitioners treat include the cough, cold, flu, diarrhea, abdominal pain, urinary tract infection, simple skin problems, menstrual problems, muscle, bone and joint pain, and many other common medical concerns. Private general practitioners generally provide more services than the public polyclinics (discussed below). For example, they make certain vaccines and aesthetic services available that the public clinics do not.

Raffles Medical Group, a major private healthcare company in Singapore, offers a range of services in its clinics, including family medical care, travel health, emergency services, minor surgery, statutory medical check ups, health screenings, x-ray services, and various specialty services, such as obstetrics and gynecology services.[2] According to the Ministry of Health, there is no data available comparing the costs of services at the private clinics to the public clinics.

Polyclinics

The public side of primary care is represented by "polyclinics," which provide 20 percent of primary level services and are highly-subsidized for patients. At this writing, there are 18 government polyclinics. An older version of the polyclinic existed well before Singapore became self-governing. By the 1920s, primary healthcare services which were provided by outpatient clinics, infant welfare clinics and traveling dispensaries.[3]

These outpatient clinics have since then been consolidated into the present-day, modern polyclinics. They provide outpatient medical care, immunization services, health screening, health education, investigative facilities, pharmacy services, and follow-up of patients discharged from hospitals. Some offer dental services as well. The average outpatient consultation fee at a polyclinic is about S$10 (see Table 6.1). This represents a subsidy of 50 percent.

Senior citizens aged above 65 years, children younger than 18, and students in school and junior colleges enjoy up to 75 percent subsidy for consultation and treatment.[4]

The polyclinics are meant to cater to lower-income Singaporeans who are unable to afford the consultation fees of private general practitioners. These generally have a longer waiting time for consultation, although they do accept walk-ins. With the recent deployment of technology, and with government efforts to revamp and upgrade the polyclinics, services are becoming much faster and more efficient. Polyclinics are most frequently located near amenities and public transportation, but, as there are only 18 polyclinics, they may be further away from patients than the more numerous general practitioner clinics.[5]

A general practitioner treats patients at a polyclinic, but several other kinds of care are available. Family Physician Clinics at the polyclinics offer consultations with doctors with qualifications in family medicine. At these Clinics, the consultations are by appointment and more time is spent with the patient. Patients with complex or multiple chronic diseases can enroll in these clinics.

A Nurse Clinician Service is also available at the polyclinics. There, senior nurses, managed by doctors, see patients whose chronic diseases are well under control.[6] Polyclinics offer basic diagnostic services, and the standard basic medication dispensed at the polyclinic pharmacies is subsidized. They also provide advice on preventive healthcare. They offer regular health talks and workshops for patient education, with the goal of increasing their level of health awareness.

Supporting the polyclinics are numerous imaging centers, laboratories (most located within the polyclinics), and mobile services.[7] Specialist

Table 6.1

FEE SCHEME
AT ANG MO KIO POLYCLINIC

General Clinic

Singapore Citizen/Adult	$9.60
Child/Elderly *	$5.40
Permanent Resident ^	$15
Non-Resident ^	$35

Family Physician Clinic

Singapore Citizen *	$24
Permanent Resident ^	$28
Non-Resident ^	$41

* Child 18 years and below. Elderly 65 years and above.

^ Includes child and elderly

Source: National Healthcare group Polyclinics [25] Our Clinics: Ang Mo Kio Polyclinic, 2011
[cited 2011 20 November]: Available from: http://www.nhgp.com.sg/ourclinics.aspx?id=32.

Outpatient Clinics, located at public hospitals, provide subsidized care on referral, either by a polyclinic or by an accident and emergency department. These clinics focus on specific medical problems and treatments such as orthopedic surgery, diabetes, eye care, head and neck surgery, etc.[8]

Up to 50 percent of subsidy is available for Singaporeans and up to 25 (as of October 2012) percent for permanent residents.[9] Specialist clinics are also located at private hospitals but are unsubsidized.

The government polyclinics are continually upgraded and expanded to keep up with the growing needs of the population. Improvements include going paperless and making records and prescriptions available electronically, use of telehealth services (for eye examinations, for instance), and automated kiosks for patient self-registration at the clinics. Studies are being done to identify service gaps and to suggest new sites for clinics that will help reduce patient travel time.[10]

Chronic Disease Management Programme

Recognizing the importance of proper management of chronic diseases, the Ministry of Health launched the Medisave for Chronic Disease Management Programme (CDMP) in 2006 to allow the use of Medisave for outpatient chronic disease care to reduce the out-of-pocket payment to encourage patients to seek timely treatment for their chronic conditions.

Under this program, patients are able to withdraw up to S$400 per year per account from their or their immediate family members' Medisave when they visit participating private general practitioners and polyclinics. In line with the principle of individual responsibility, patients are required to pay the first S$30 of the bill (as the deductible) as well as 15 percent of the balance of the bill (as co-insurance).

Diabetes mellitus was the only condition covered under the scheme when the program was first launched in 2006. Over time, more and more diseases were added. The chronic diseases now covered are asthma, diabetes, hypertension, lipid disorders, stroke, chronic obstructive pulmonary disease, schizophrenia, major depression, dementia, and bipolar disorder.

This scheme is complemented by the Community Health Assist Scheme (which provides portable subsidies) at private general practitioner clinics.

Community Health Assist Scheme

Increasingly, the public system has been forging ties with the large networks of private general practitioners, who are being enlisted to provide basic care, treat certain chronic illnesses, and provide dental care. Formerly called the Primary Care Partnership Scheme but renamed the Community Health Assist Scheme, the program was introduced in 2000 and is targeted at lower-income and disabled elderly Singaporeans. They can receive subsidized outpatient services, including dental services, at the private clinics just as they would at a government polyclinic. Raffles Medical Clinics, for example, are accredited for the program.[11]

The program also covers treatment of common chronic diseases under CDMP. A survey conducted in 2010 had revealed that, on a per doctor basis, polyclinics were treating a disproportionately high number of chronic disease cases. It was determined that polyclinics alone would not be able to meet the long-term, increasing demand, thus, the program was expanded to allow for the treatment of more chronic diseases at private clinics.[12]

In order to allow more patients to benefit from the program, the cut-off income limit to qualify for subsidies has been raised from S$800 to S$1,500 per capita monthly household income (which is the median level) and the qualifying age has been lowered from 65 to 40 years.

The relative ease of getting treatment at a nearby private general practitioner at subsidized prices is a motivation for patients, especially those requiring chronic disease management to get proper and timely treatment. Patients can withdraw money from their Medisave accounts to pay for these treatments, thereby reducing their out-of-pocket expenditures. Currently, patients can use up to ten Medisave accounts (their own and their families') up to S$400 per account per year. Each claim is subject to a deductible of S$30 and a 15 percent co-payment.[13]

As I write in early 2012, the government is developing a masterplan to broaden and deepen the current public–private partnership. The goal is to enhance the treatment of chronic disease by bringing together private general practitioners with other healthcare professionals (for example, nurses, and allied health professionals) to form a team approach to care. Preliminary ideas under consideration include: Community Health Centres to provide ancillary support services to the general practitioners, including laboratory tests, radiologic services, podiatry, physiotherapy, care coordination, dietetics, and retinal examination; Family Medicine Clinics that would bring together private general practitioners and allied medical professionals under one roof, with more supportive services available onsite; Medical Centres, where ambulatory procedures (for example, day surgery for cataract removal) can be carried out in the community. It would also allow the general practitioners to work with specialists to co-manage patients with complex disease conditions.[14]

Other Public–Private Partnerships

Another public–private partnership worth noting is the work of the National Kidney Foundation (NKF) of Singapore and its approach to kidney disease, specifically end-stage renal disease where the kidneys no longer function correctly and dialysis or a transplant is necessary. NKF is engaged in public education, screening, and operates a network of centers to deal with the disease.[15]

The National Kidney Foundation has been able to establish partnerships and sponsorships with corporations and has built a network of 24 dialysis centers across Singapore. It performs home visits to help patients with peritoneal dialysis, a home-based therapy. It also offers its services to companies, such as performing health screenings to employees for conditions that may lead to kidney diseases.[16]

It has been estimated that the NKF treats over 70 percent of patients with end-stage renal disease and continues to expand its work in preventing the disease.[17]

Hospitals and Higher Levels of Care

I wrote earlier that private practitioners handle 80 percent of primary care attendances and public polyclinics 20 percent. The numbers reverse themselves in the secondary and tertiary care areas (defined as specialist care, advanced medical investigation and treatment), where 80 percent of inpatient care is provided by the public sector and 20 percent by private. Eight public hospitals and several national specialty centers provide the bulk of all care.[18] In all, there were 30 hospitals in Singapore in 2010, with 15 in the private sector (albeit of smaller sizes) and 15 in the public sector.[19] The public hospitals contained almost 8,900 beds while the private hospitals had just over 2,600 beds.[20] Also in 2010, 80 percent of hospitalizations were in the public sector and 20 percent in the private sector.

Patients are free to use either the public or private system, according to their willingness and ability to pay. Public hospitals are obliged care regardless of ability of pay. No proof of ability to pay is required before admission to public hospitals. According to the Ministry of Health, there is no measurable difference in outcomes between the two systems. Private hospitals serve a sizeable number of foreigners as well as Singaporeans. The private sector offers additional services in their hospitals that some patients may be looking for and which are unavailable in the subsidized ward classes in the public sector. Parkway Pantai and Raffles Medical Group are two of the leading private hospital care providers in Singapore. The United States'

Johns Hopkins University has established a small medical center in the country. Generally, private sector hospitals provide more choice to consumers who are willing to spend more, demand faster services, and seek more amenities. Luxury-level amenities are available in some hospitals. Private hospitals are more involved in medical tourism than are the public hospitals. In time, private hospitals will play a greater role in the public system as the government plans to tap into their spare capacity to treat some of its subsidized patients. Bed occupancy rates in the private hospitals average about 55 percent.[21] Right now, for example, National University Hospital is renting 30 beds at West Point Hospital, a private acute and convalescent hospital in Singapore, and has been doing so since 2009.

Public Hospital Infrastructure

Soon after independence, the government began upgrading the hospitals, which had been built before the Second World War, and acquiring modern equipment. It decided to invest in the public hospitals and take the lead in improving care because it judged the private sector unable to develop sophisticated specialties due to the high costs involved. Hospitals were upgraded gradually, beginning with the Singapore General Hospital in the late 1970s, with others following suit. New hospitals also began to be built as the government saw increases in the general population, with a tertiary specialist hospital upgraded in 1985, and a secondary care hospital in 2010 due to the increasing need for elderly care. Two more hospitals are being built to address the increased demand of the aging population. One, being built in the western part of Singapore, is slated to open in 2014 with a 700-bed capacity. Another, serving the residents in northeast Singapore, will be built by 2018.[22]

The infrastructure improvements continue, serving to show the continual efforts on the part of the government to be prepared for the challenges that changing times demand. Healthcare Budget 2011 provides for a number of facilities at major public hospitals to be upgraded. The Budget also unveiled the government's plans to develop new intermediate- and long-term care facilities to meet the growing needs of the elderly. The plans involve building community hospitals, expanding nursing home capacities, and building new nursing homes.

Delivery of Hospital Care

Care is delivered at general, regional hospitals, with more specialized care at the National Centres. The general hospitals offer acute inpatient services, specialist outpatient services, and a 24-hour emergency department. In 2010, there were over 11,000 beds (combined public and private sectors) in 30 hospitals (15 public and 15 private, including specialty centers, community hospitals, and chronic sick hospitals).[23] The average length of stay in the acute care hospitals, according to the Ministry of Health, was about five days, and the average occupancy rate was about 75 percent. According to information gathered in a parliamentary question and answer session, in 2010 there were four million outpatient attendances at the public hospitals, with two-thirds of them subsidized. Government subsidy to public hospitals for patients totaled just under S$2.25 billion, and most of the public hospitals ran at 85 percent capacity on average.[24]

National Specialty Centres

Along with the hospitals providing general care, Singapore has developed a number of organizations that focus on medical specialties, including cancer, oral care, cardiovascular disease, diseases of the nervous system, and skin diseases. The National Heart Centre, as an example, is a facility with just under 200 beds that handles over 9,000 inpatient admissions each year. Offering a full range of treatment from preventative to rehabilitative, it is the national and regional referral center for any cardiovascular complications. Research, teaching, and training are also conducted there. By way of contrast, the National Skin Centre provides dermatological services on an outpatient basis. It also conducts research and aids in the training of medical students.[25]

Intermediate and Long-Term Care

Intermediate and long-term care services are delivered through private sector as well as voluntary welfare groups. A number of home-based and center-based options are available to the sick and elderly, so that they can be taken care of in a comfortable and familiar environment in their own community. These include community hospitals, chronic sick hospitals, nursing homes, and hospices.[26] These organizations generally are not designed to offer the highest levels of technology and critical care available at the general hospitals. To encourage community participation and initiative in providing care to the elderly, chronically sick, terminally ill, and mentally ill, the government began to provide subsidies to some private institutions and Voluntary Welfare Organizations providing such care, and continues to do so today.

An array of services is available to patients depending on their needs (see Table 6.2). With the increasing numbers of elderly people in the population and the demand for these services escalating, this area is receiving more attention and funding from the government. For example, in mid-2011, the Ministry of Health announced plans to recruit and retain more staff for this sector through a pilot central employment initiative. Under the program, professionals, including physiotherapists, occupational therapists, and speech therapists, would be recruited and deployed.[27]

Dental Services

Individuals can have their dental needs taken care of at specially-designated polyclinics and hospitals and at the National Dental Centre. Schoolchildren are provided dental services through 200 clinics located in schools and via 30 mobile clinics. Under the Community Health Assist Scheme, Singaporeans who qualify can receive subsidies for selected dental services at the private participating dental clinics.[28]

Oversight Management

The Ministry of Health, with its statutory boards, regulates both the private and public sectors. One board, the Health Sciences Authority, is tasked with monitoring and ensuring the safety of health-related products. Another, the Health Promotion Board, undertakes national health promotion and disease prevention efforts.[29]

The Ministry licenses all hospitals, clinics, clinical laboratories, nursing homes, and other healthcare institutes in Singapore. A record of all the medical practitioners is maintained at the Singapore Medical Council, a statutory board operating under the Ministry of Health. Within the council's purview also lies the task of governance, regulation of professional conduct, and ethics of the registered doctors.[30] Various professional bodies, including the Singapore Dental Council, Singapore Nursing Board, and Singapore Pharmacy Council, regulate the other healthcare professions.

The Cluster System

All of Singapore's public healthcare institutions and facilities belong to a government holding company called MOH Holdings and are divided into six clusters, each anchored by a regional hospital. As of this writing, the new organization is almost complete, with some elements still evolving, according

Table 6.2

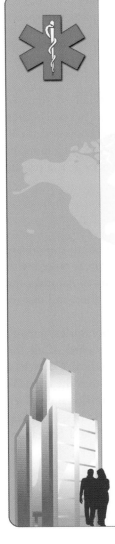

INTERMEDIATE AND LONG-TERM CARE (ILTC) SERVICES

Community-based ILTC Services

1. Home-based
- Home Medical
- Home Nursing
- Home Hospice Care Services

2. Centre-based
- Day Rehabilitation Centres for the Elderly
- Dementia Day Care Centres
- Psychiatric Day Care Centres
- Psychiatric Rehabilitation Homes

Residential ILTC Services

1. Community Hospitals

2. Chronic Sick Hospitals

3. Nursing Homes
- Voluntary Welfare Organizations (VWO) Nursing Homes receiving MOH subsidies
- VWO Nursing Homes not receiving MOH subsidies
- Private Nursing Homes under MOH portable subsidy scheme
- Private Nursing Homes not under MOH portable subsidy scheme

4. Inpatient Hospices

5. Sheltered Home for Ex-Mentally ill

6. Respite Care

Source: Ministry of Health (MOH) Singapore [27] Intermediate and Long-Term Care (ILTC) Services. 2011 [cited 10 November 2011];
Available from:
http://www.moh.gov.sg/content/moh_web/home/our_healthcare_system/
Healthcare_Services/Intermediate_And_Long-Term_Care_Residential.html.

to the Ministry of Health. For example, decisions regarding which polyclinics and step-down facilities are organized under which tertiary care hospitals are still in the process of being made.

Once a dormant holding company, MOH Holdings has evolved into a high-level, active umbrella organization that provides strategic direction, facilitates cooperation across the clusters, and ensures that the Ministry of Health's goals and priorities are realized throughout the system. Among its many current specific initiatives are: developing a national information technology framework for healthcare; providing for joint recruitment of care professionals; and developing a talent management and human resources framework for the entire system. The Permanent Secretary of the Ministry of Health chairs MOH Holdings.[31]

At one time, Singapore's public sector healthcare institutions were divided into two broad clusters, one that included National University Hospital and the other Singapore General Hospital. It was thought that this organization would encourage competition between the two groups, allow for greater integration of care within each, and promote economies of scale. As of early 2012, as mentioned above, a structural transformation is taking place that reorganizes care into six regional groups in an effort to respond to the needs of the growing number of older patients with complex, chronic diseases. Each cluster is anchored by a regional hospital that continues to provide acute care, but with tight linkage to specialty centers, tertiary care hospitals, intermediate and long-term care facilities, and polyclinics and general practitioner clinics that are not publically owned.

The regional hospitals will offer the acute care that they excel at delivering. Illnesses that require a higher level of care would be referred to one of the five National Centres (devoted to eye, skin, dental, cancer, and heart care), or to one of two hospitals offering comprehensive specialty care, each of which, in turn, is closely tied in to a medical school. The close association of these hospitals with the schools and their environment of research, innovation, and continual improvement, will be to the benefit of patients.

The many various intermediate and long-term care institutions also residing within each cluster provide the necessary services for moving stabilized chronic disease patients away from hospitalization and acute care to a more appropriate and less critical level of care. The Agency for Integrated Care helps ensure that the transitions of patients to lower levels of care happen smoothly and are appropriate for the individual situation.[32] In this way, patients can receive continued treatment and monitoring in the most convenient setting conducive for their recovery.

Diabetes patients, to mention just one example, would benefit greatly from a cluster system like Singapore's. According to the 2010 National Health Survey, over 11 percent of the population between aged 18 and 69 years suffer from the disease, making it a major healthcare challenge in Singapore.[33] The disease can be effectively controlled through a diligent and regular application of medication, diet, exercise, and regular check ups. Yet it is estimated that only a small percentage of sufferers keeps the disease under control. Individuals cite reasons such as lack of time or distance to be traveled for medical appointments, no caregiver at home, and a lack of motivation, among others.

The cluster system would allow diabetes patients and their medical records, through the electronic health record system, to move smoothly through various levels of care from acute care, as necessary, at their regional hospital, to step-down care at a nearby intermediate or long-term care facility, and finally to a local, neighborhood polyclinic, where regular appointments for check ups and regular treatment could easily be scheduled and taken. If complications occur, they would be quickly detected, and patients could be efficiently moved back up the system to the regional hospital, for instance, for acute care.

The government is also giving private general practitioners a role to play in the cluster system. With about 2,000 practitioners located in communities throughout Singapore, their facilities are far more numerous than the polyclinics and are usually located much closer to potential patients. Thus they generally offer more convenience to the patient, including less travel time and difficulty. This deepening of the private–public relationship again illustrates the government's continuing efforts to innovate, to better itself, and to improve the quality of its patients' experiences.

***

Chapter 6: KEY POINTS

- Primary care is provided mainly by approximately 2,000 private general practitioners in Singapore
  - Public facilities available for primary care are called polyclinics and are multi-doctor facilities with support services and often laboratories on the premises. The polyclinics account for 20 percent of primary care attendances
  - There are 18 polyclinics in the system, and they are highly subsidized for eligible patients

- Under the Community Health Assist Scheme, private doctors are being enlisted to provide basic care, treat certain chronic illnesses, and provide dental care
  - Visits are subsidized for the lower-income and disabled
  - The Scheme helps to alleviate the very high patient load at the polyclinics

- Higher levels of care are provided mainly by the public hospitals, although private hospitals exist as well.
  - There are 15 public and 15 private hospitals in Singapore
  - The public Specialty Centres offer focused care for cancer, heart disease, and other illnesses

- Intermediate or long-term care is provided by a variety of institutions including community hospitals, chronic sick hospitals, nursing homes, and hospices

- Singapore is reorganizing its hospitals and all other care facilities into six regionally-oriented public healthcare "clusters"
  - Each cluster is anchored by a general hospital

CHAPTER 7

Investing in the Future through Medical Education and Research

Education, research, innovation, and continual improvement are fundamental to the success of the Singapore healthcare system. The government has two broad goals in mind as it directs investment into healthcare knowledge and medical research. One is to better serve the people of Singapore, making certain the healthcare system is staffed with highly-competent, highly-trained doctors, nurses, and other medical personnel, and that the system is as effective and efficient as it can possibly be by incorporating relevant new technologies and research findings in the delivery of care. The other is to make economic progress in Singapore by developing the country into a world-class research center, attracting corporations to its laboratories, inviting collaboration with the private sector in an effort to bring innovations to the market, and supporting new Singapore-based companies in the technology or biomedical industries.

Medical Education and Training

There is a widely acknowledged shortage of doctors and other healthcare professionals in Singapore, currently with 18 doctors per 10,000 population.[1] The Ministry of Health estimates that growth in demand for medical professionals will increase about 50% between 2012 and 2020, requiring some 20,000 professionals: doctors, nurses, dentists, pharmacists and allied health professionals. Some observers believe the shortage of doctors is a major challenge that must be addressed through new ways of education and training—with the traditional apprentice method and emphasis on examinations in need of change.[2]

Aside from the increase in students being trained in the local universities, as discussed below, the government allows foreign-trained doctors whose degrees are recognized by Singapore to practice in the country. Other health workers are "imported" as well, both to meet domestic demand and to provide care to medical tourists.[3]

The Singapore system includes two undergraduate medical schools and one postgraduate medical school. The oldest medical school, part of the National University of Singapore, maintains a traditional European approach based on the British model to training doctors; the postgraduate medical school, a collaboration between NUS and Duke University, offers an American-style approach and prepares its graduates to be clinician-scientists. The third and newest, part of the Nanyang Technological University, will train doctors with an innovative curriculum developed in conjunction with the Imperial College London, combining science, technology, and business management.

Yong Loo Lin School of Medicine

NUS's medical school, now known as the Yong Loo Lin School of Medicine, was founded in 1905 as the "Straits Settlements and Federated Malay States Government Medical School." The school's name was changed to King Edward VII Medical School in 1912, when the King Edward VII Memorial Fund made a gift of S$120,000 to the school. Recognition for the school's License in Medicine and Surgery came in 1916 from the General Medical Council of Great Britain. It was absorbed as the Faculty of Medicine of the University of Malaya, an early precursor of the National University of Singapore, in 1949.

In 2005, the school became the Yong Loo Lin School of Medicine after being given a gift of S$100 million by the Yong Loo Lin Trust with the intent to boost development of multidisciplinary translational research pertinent to Singapore's health needs.

In 2008, the School of Medicine, with the National University Hospital and the Faculty of Dentistry, came together under the common governance of the National University Health System. This change in governance was effected to make possible better synergy between education, research, and clinical care.[4]

The School is modeled after the British approach to undergraduate medical studies and graduate students with a Bachelor of Medicine and a Bachelor of Surgery. A Bachelor degree in Nursing is also offered. Graduate programs include Masters of Medicine in numerous specialties; Masters and

PhDs in various biomedical disciplines, and the Master of Nursing degree. In 2011, the Yong Loo Lin School of Medicine was ranked as the top medical school in Asia and 18th in the world overall by QS World University Rankings by Subject (Medicine).[5]

Academic departments include the following: Alice Lee Centre for Nursing Studies, anesthesia, anatomy, biochemistry, epidemiology and public health, diagnostic radiology, medicine, microbiology, obstetrics and gynecology, ophthalmology, orthopedic surgery, otolaryngology, pediatrics, pathology, pharmacology, physiology, psychological medicine, and surgery. The school operates several centers for advanced education and research, as follows: Centre for Biomedical Ethics, Centre for Molecular Epidemiology, Centre for Environmental and Occupational Health Research, Centre for Health Policy and Management, Singapore Epidemiology of Eye Diseases Centre (also known as SEED), Centre for Translational Medicine, although some of these centers will be moved under the School of Public Health.

The school admits fewer than 300 students in each class. In 2011, 255 Bachelor degrees were conferred along with numerous Master degrees (see Figure 7.1 for more details). Its course of study is a five-year program emphasizing the clinical side of medicine. Its seven areas of focus are cancer, cardiovascular disease, aging and the neurosciences, gastrointestinal and liver disease, immunology, regenerative medicine, and infectious diseases, all conditions common in Singapore's population.[6] The Centre for Nursing Studies graduated 53 students with the Bachelor's degree and 22 students with the Master of Nursing degree in 2011.

The school also offers an extensive list of graduate programs. Degrees include Doctor of Philosophy (School of Medicine), Doctor of Philosophy (Cancer Science Institute), Doctor of Philosophy (Nursing), Doctor of Philosophy (Joint PhD with Imperial College), Master of Science (School of Medicine), Master of Science (Nursing), and Master of Clinical Investigation. It also offers a Master of Medicine degree in the following concentrations: Anesthesiology, Diagnostic Radiology, Emergency Medicine, Family Medicine, Internal Medicine, Obstetrics and Gynecology, Ophthalmology, Orthopedic Surgery, Otorhinolaryngology, Pediatric Medicine, Psychiatry, and Surgery. The school's executive and professional staff numbers almost 250 (see Figure 7.1).

Associated with the Yong Loo Lin School is NUS's Health Cluster at the Faculty of Arts and Social Sciences. The Health Cluster is made up of almost 30 faculty members from many different departments in the Arts and Social Sciences faculty, including Communications and New Media, Economics, Geography, Japanese Studies, Psychology, Sociology, and Social

Figure 7.1

NUS YONG LOO LIN SCHOOL OF MEDICINE

Class Of 2011

255	Bachelor's Degree conferred
9	Master of Clinical Investigation Degrees conferred
164	Master of Medicine Degrees conferred
18	Master of Public Health Degrees conferred
27	Master of Science Degrees conferred
7	Master of Science in infectious Diseases, Vaccinology and Drug Discovery (Joint MSc with Basel) Degrees conferred
18	Master of Science in Speech & Language Pathology Degrees conferred
65	Doctoral Degrees conferred

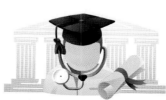

Faculty and Staff 2011

242	Executive and Professional staff
447	Non-academic staff
546	Other teaching staff
473	Research staff
258	Academic staff

NUS FACULTY OF DENTISTRY

Class Of 2011

42	Bachelor's Degree conferred
5	Graduate Diplomas awarded
11	Master Degrees conferred
4	Doctoral Degrees (Research) conferred

Faculty and Staff 2011

8	Executive and Professional staff
42	Non-academic staff
8	Research staff
32	Academic staff
2	Visiting staff

NUS ALICE LEE CENTRE FOR NURSING STUDIES

Class Of 2011

53	Bachelor's Degree conferred (18 Honours)
22	Master of Nursing Degrees conferred

Faculty and Staff 2011

6	Executive and Professional staff
10	Non-academic staff
2	Visiting teaching staff
8	Research staff
28	Academic staff

Work. The group is committed to faculty and graduate student research into health-related issues important to Singapore and the region.[7]

Reflecting its membership, the Cluster's research projects are multi-disciplinary and include cross-campus collaborations with the Yong Loo Lin School of Medicine and the Faculties of Law, Business, and Engineering. Areas of research include: health policy, long-term healthcare financing, addiction behavior, neuropsychology, disease pandemics, and post-disaster health risks. In the area of aging, work is being done on issues such as active aging, social isolation and health, care-giving, and end-of-life.

The Cluster also supports health research by graduate students. According to its website, the group has graduate students conducting research in fertility, mortality, public health, HIV, and aging, using data from Singapore and other parts of Asia.[8]

Duke-NUS Graduate Medical School

Duke University of the United States and the National University of Singapore collaborated to found this graduate medical school—known as Duke-NUS—with its orientation on biomedical sciences. It was established as part of Singapore's strategy to become a leading hub for biomedical research and education for the purpose of training medical professionals who would be able to support the biomedical initiative. Duke and NUS formalized their arrangement in 2005, and the first class of 26 medical students entered the school in June of 2007. It now admits over 50 students each year.

The school follows the American model of medical education in that students must first complete their undergraduate degrees before entering the school, where they will typically earn their MDs in four years. The school also offers a PhD and a combined MD/PhD program for students intent on pursuing a biomedical-research-oriented clinical practice and which may take as long as seven years to complete.

The Duke-NUS curriculum is patterned after Duke University's Medical School and represents a shift away from the classical method of educating doctors by lectures and clinic ward experience. At Duke-NUS, a more active and collaborative type of training takes place. It emphasizes creative thinking skills and problem-solving over pure memorization.

A team-based learning approach and problem-based learning strategies are used in the medical education process. Small-group and collaborative learning are the norm. The school's cooperative team-based learning approach is based on a model developed by Larry Michaelsen, a Professor of Management at the University of Central Missouri in the United States.

Traditional lectures are converted into voice-annotated presentations that the students review prior to class. Required readings and the review of all lecture material on a given topic also take place before class. The class (divided into student teams) then focuses on assuring understanding and problem-solving by principle application with the help of the faculty. The faculty itself is multidisciplinary and consists of teams of clinicians and scientists supported by education faculty with expertise in the science of learning. The aim is to have the classroom discussions driven by student enquiry rather than faculty answers or lecturing. The classes include activities that require students to apply problem-solving and to make meaningful choices to respond to the challenges. Students are given feedback from their peers as well as from the faculty. Useful social media tools such as Facebook are integrated into all aspects of learning.

According to Frank Starmer, Associate Dean for Learning Technologies at the school, "by design, from the beginning, we avoided silos by not having traditional departments. Our current organization facilitates cross discipline interaction. Professor Ranga Krishnan's leadership (he is Dean of the medical school), has moved us forward with innovative approaches to learning, clinical care and outreach. Said another way, our organization is simply fun to be part of. We are not aligned with a departmental organization. We have four divisions: Education, Research, Admin, Clinical Sciences."[9]

Associate Dean Starmer has emphasized the importance of stimulating students' curiosity—even a "childish curiosity"—and imagination, as he sees those as key components to problem-solving. He prefers student-centric learning and even endeavors to rekindle the joy of leaning in school.[10]

In addition to the MD, the school offers a PhD Program in Integrated Biology and Medicine. The program emphasizes training in translational science. Specialty tracks are offered in cancer and stem cell biology, cardiovascular and metabolic disorders, neuroscience and behavioral disorders, health services and systems research, and emerging infectious diseases. The school also offers a combined MD/PhD program for students pursuing research-oriented careers, combining biomedical research with the practice of clinical medicine.

Duke-NUS specialty centers for advanced scientific research and education include Center for Quantitative Medicine, The Cognitive Neuroscience Laboratory, and The Lien Centre for Palliative Care.

As of this writing, Duke-NUS has more than 500 full-time and adjunct faculty in research and education; has received approximately S$120 million in research funding; and participates in more than 35 research collaborations and research partnerships. In addition, 18 patent applications have been filed, and one biotech company has been founded by two members of the faculty.[11] These two medical schools are closely aligned with tertiary hospitals—Duke-NUS with the Singapore General Hospital and the Yong Loo Lin School of Medicine with the National University Hospital. The linkage brings these institutions together in an environment conducive for research and development, innovation, and high-quality training.

Singapore's Newest Medical School

The Lee Kong Chian School of Medicine is scheduled to begin training its first class of 50 students in 2013. When fully realized, the school plans to admit 150 students each year. The School is a partnership of the Nanyang Technological University (NTU) and Imperial College London, and faculty will be drawn from Imperial College as well as recruited from Singapore and around the world.

The NTU approach to medical education will be forward-looking as healthcare in the future increasingly will be built at the intersection of medicine and science and technology. The school will train new generations of physicians with a new curriculum bringing together the "strength of Imperial College's world-leading medical expertise with NTU's core strengths in engineering and business," according to Dr. Su Guaning, former President of Nanyang Technological University. The School will start out "not just training the best clinicians but also make a deep impact on the innovation of medical devices and the healthcare system as a whole." Interdisciplinary learning will include the engineering behind new medical devices, health economics, and management skills at Nanyang Business School.

It is to be an undergraduate medical program taking five years with the awarding of a joint Imperial College–Nanyang Technological University Bachelor of Medicine and Bachelor of Surgery. Faculty members will be drawn from Imperial College London, as well as recruited from Singapore and around the world.

The School plans to enroll the best students who also show an ability to become caring doctors committed to serving the community. Testing and interviewing of prospective students are meant "to identify the most capable students who have the best chance of becoming the patient-centered doctors that you and I would want to have caring for us," according to Senior Vice Dean, Professor Martyn Partridge.[12]

Clinical training will take place in conjunction with the National Healthcare Group as well as other hospitals, and will give students exposure to a range of healthcare settings, including polyclinics, acute care hospitals, and national specialty centers.[13]

Continuing Education of Medical Personnel

In order to upgrade doctors' clinical capabilities and knowledge, many would have gone through the Ministry of Health's Health Manpower Development Programme training, an overseas skills-based attachment program in selected overseas institutions. Doctors also need to undergo compulsory Continuing Medical Education (CME) in programs approved by the Singapore Medical Council in order to keep abreast of the advances in the medical field. Since 2005, all fully and conditionally registered doctors must meet CME requirements before their practicing certificates are renewed. Doctors earn Continuing Medical Education "points" by attending or participating in approved programs and events, publishing in journals, self-study and online programs, and earning overseas postgraduate degrees or diplomas.[14]

Members of the Academy of Medicine Singapore, College of Family Physicians Singapore, Singapore Medical Association, as well as doctors working in both the public and private sectors are represented on a committed that accredits CME programs and reviews CME policies and programs.[15]

Nanyang Technological University

As a leading science and technology university, NTU conducts a broad range of research, including biomedical engineering and computational biology. The College of Engineering is home to the School of Chemical and Biomedical Engineering, which conducts research in many areas, including nanotechnology with a focus on health, chemical process engineering with application to the pharmaceutical industries, nanomedicine and biomedical devices for improving healthcare, and biomolecular engineering with a noteworthy focus on biomedicine and small molecule anticancer drugs.

The College of Science contains the School of Biological Sciences with two areas of prime investigation: structural biology/biochemistry and also molecular genetics/cell biology. Research areas include, among others, genomics, cell biology, molecular biology, infectious disease and immunology. The University also houses a large number of research centers working in numerous areas of inquiry. A few of them, relevant to healthcare, include bioinformatics, bionanosystems, and structural biology.[16]

The Saw Swee Hock School of Public Health

The origins of public health research and teaching in Singapore can be traced back to the establishment of the Department of Social Medicine and Public Health in the then King Edward VII College of Medicine in 1948. Much has changed since then and the Department's focus has reflected the changing landscape of public health in Singapore. From involvement in the Singapore Cancer Registry to pioneering etiological research on high incidence cancers in Singapore, it was renamed the Department of Community Occupational and Family Medicine in 1987, and expanded its research to include epidemiology of cardiovascular and eye diseases, development of monitoring standards for environmental carcinogens and population-based cohort studies.

Responding to an increased need for public health training, the Department converted the Master of Medicine Programme to the Master of Public Health degree in 2007. Two years later, the Department became the Department of Epidemiology and Public Health at the National University of Singapore. These changes precipitated expansion into new areas of research, including the genetic determinants of disease in Asian populations, the mathematical and statistical modeling of infectious disease epidemiology, as well as the role of gene environment interactions in shaping chronic disease risk factors in the Singapore population.

The Department of Epidemiology and Public Health was transformed in 2011 into a new school of public health, the Saw Swee Hock School of Public Health. The unique character of the School is reflected in two of its goals. The first is how to reduce the cost of healthcare spending in Singapore now that most traditional public health issues are well met by the current system. The School plans to use extensive quantitative modeling to understand potential consequences of Singapore's current health policies as well as any proposed changes, allowing for very realistic conceptual experimentation. The second goal is to become a regional leader in South and Southeast Asia health policy.

The School will train the nation's future leaders in healthcare and will perform research into and develop new models of public health and care delivery. It aims to strengthen the teaching of undergraduate medical students at the Yong Loo Lin School of Medicine and intensify research efforts in chronic non-communicable diseases such as diabetes, hypertension, cancer and heart disease. The School also plans to develop strong infectious diseases capabilities and help Singapore be well-prepared for potential new epidemics in the future. It offers a Master in Public Health that can be pursued on a full-time or part-time basis. At this time of writing, specializations are available in clinical epidemiology, global health, and occupational and environmental health.[17]

The School is organized into four domain areas: Epidemiology—focusing on cancer, cardiovascular and metabolic diseases, nutritional epidemiology, eye disease and infectious diseases, and new areas of research such as mathematical modeling and surveillance of infectious diseases; Biostatistics—health statistics and analysis plus newer areas of research including public health genomics; Health Systems and Policy Research—research initiatives that include utilizing mathematical and econometric modeling for policy decision-making as well as the development of new health monitoring devices; and Health Behaviour and Health Promotion—focused on behavior change interventions, with research aimed at reducing high-risk sexual behavior as well as workplace health promotion interventions for an aging population. Since 2011, the School and the London School of Hygiene and Tropical Medicine have been collaborating on public health research and education.[18]

According to Professor Chia Kee Seng, Dean, Saw Swee Hock School of Public Health, the School will be active in health education and promotion, health systems and policy, looking at questions such as how to model care systems for outbreaks. He sees disease prevention to be of primary importance and is committed to finding ways to promote prevention—especially of diseases such as diabetes—including helping the people of Singapore eat better, healthier foods.

Singapore's Policy Research Centers

The Saw Swee Hock School of Public Health is not alone in the investigation and research into healthcare policy. Singapore is investing in all kinds of policy research—organized inquiries into areas of importance to the country and the region, including education, the economy, urban issues, national defense, and more. Below I discuss a number of policy institutes located in Singapore along with a description of their special areas of interest.

Lee Kuan Yew School of Public Policy

The Lee Kuan Yew School of Public Policy at the National University of Singapore is led by Kishore Mahbubani, Dean and Professor in the Practice of Public Policy. The school is dedicated to the education and training of the emerging generation of Asian policymakers and leaders. Its aim is to "raise the standards of governance throughout the region, improve the lives of the region's people and, in so doing, contribute to the transformation of Asia."

It has formed partnerships with the John F. Kennedy School of Government at Harvard University, Columbia University's School of International and Public Affairs, the London School of Economics and Political Science, and the Institut d'Études Politiques de Paris.

The School offers one PhD and four Masters programs: the Master in Public Policy, the Master in Public Administration, the Master in Public Management, and the Master in Public Administration and Management. It also offers the Doctor of Philosophy in Public Policy, with specialization in development studies, economic policy, international relations and security, social and environmental policy, and public management and governance.[19] The School currently has 400 students from approximately 50 nations.

The Lee Kuan Yew School of Public Policy has established a number of research centers that bring together leading academics, international thinkers, politicians and others to study and discourse upon topics important to Asia's future. The research centers are: Asia Competitiveness Institute, Centre for Asia and Globalisation, Institute of Policy Studies, and Institute of Water Policy.[20]

Initiative to Improve Health in Asia

Led by the National University of Singapore, the Initiative to Improve Health in Asia—known as NIHA—is dedicated to improving public health and healthcare delivery in Asia. NIHA focuses on high-level thinking and policy formulation in public health and health systems development in Asia, and it seeks to make Singapore a leader in healthcare policy and healthcare research. NIHA is coordinated by the NUS Global Asia Institute, in collaboration with the Lee Kuan Yew School of Public Policy, Yong Loo Lin School of Medicine, and the National University of Singapore Business School.[21]

NIHA's research encompasses medical, economic, social, and ethical issues in all aspects of healthcare, including organization, financing, management and delivery of care. Priority is given to important, relevant issues in Asia; for example, the growing percentage of elderly people in the population. NIHA seeks out research partners across Asia to help it in its work. It also organizes forums on health policy, one recent one being "Combating Chronic Disease in Asia—Gaps and Innovations." The forums attempt to encourage consensus-building and partnerships among healthcare policymakers and industry leaders. NIHA's leadership program is a two-week-long program aimed at training future leaders in the healthcare sector. Topics in the most recent leadership program included health policy and program design, implementation and evaluation, and healthcare leadership and management, and was aimed at emerging leaders contributing to the healthcare field.[22]

Global Asia Institute

Global Asia Institute operates within the National University of Singapore, and University President Tan Chorh Chuan has said that through the Institute's works, the University expects to become "a pre-eminent center for thought-leadership, research and education on critical issues for Asia."[23]

The Institute's mission is to lead in research and scholarship directed toward topics vital to Asia's future. It takes a "holistic" approach to addressing Asian issues and draws upon many areas of knowledge at the University, from engineering and design to social sciences and public policy. It also works in collaboration with scholars and research/policy centers internationally.

The Institute specializes in the large, fundamental issues important to Singapore, Asia, and the world. Current areas being investigated include: challenges in the global economy; the future of urban societies; and managing resources for livable cities.[24]

Institute for Policy Studies

The Institute for Policy Studies is a think-tank dedicated to the research and analysis of domestic policy issues. Its research is primarily focused on Singapore-centric subjects, but it also keeps an international perspective because of Singapore's interconnectedness to global economics and politics. Major areas of research include: Arts, Culture, and Media; Demography and Family; Economics and Business; Politics and Governance; Society and Identity.

Examples of the Institute's work within these areas include: artistic freedom, development of creative industries, old and new rules for evolving internet media (Arts, Culture, and Media); causes and consequences of Singapore's low total fertility rate and policy responses, the characteristics of the aging population and the needs and support systems required for the older citizens and residents, and immigration and labor mobility policies (Demography and Family).

While most of the Institute's projects deal with current concerns, there are also long-term studies contemplating future developments in Singapore.[25]

Science and Technology Research in Singapore—A*STAR

Singapore's Agency for Science, Technology and Research—A*STAR—is an important player in science and technology research with a worldwide reputation. It strives to turn research into practical products, services, and businesses that will benefit the nation's economy and build its reputation as a world-class research and development center. Its goal is to accelerate "the translation of research findings" into commercial products and services that will benefit Singapore's economy. The agency supports key industries important to Singapore's economy by promoting manpower training and development in the sciences, engineering, and technology; undertaking research and development through its research institutes; and promoting commercial application of scientific knowledge and technology advances through collaboration with industry and commercialization of intellectual property. Its efforts to improve the economy of Singapore through health technologies include encouraging foreign companies and medical device firms to set up shop in Singapore, and also starting companies itself.

Singapore is fortunate that all the country's major investment decisions, finance, foreign relations and politics, and economic development issues are addressed through a centralized cabinet process. As it became apparent to government leaders that Singapore might thrive as a science and technology based economy, a number of scientific research institutes were created in areas such as molecular and cell biology, clinical sciences, and medical biology. Eventually, A*STAR became the parent overseer of these institutes and was placed under the guidance of the former head of the Economic Development Board who had been instrumental in restructuring the manufacturing sector.[26] The Agency includes 14 biomedical and physical sciences and engineering research institutes and six consortia and centers, located in Biopolis, Fusionopolis, a world-class science and engineering research complex, and in the immediate area.

Under A*STAR's aegis are a number of organizations that oversee different sectors of research and development, including, Biomedical Research Council; Science and Engineering Research Council; and the A*STAR Joint Council.

The Biomedical Research Council oversees the development of Singapore's core research capabilities in bioprocessing, chemical synthesis, and genomics, among many other areas of scientific inquiry. The Council also promotes translational medicine and cross-disciplinary research in the healthcare area, in collaboration with the Ministry of Health, and supports biomedical research in the wider scientific community such as public universities and hospitals.

The Science and Engineering Research Council's purview is physical sciences and engineering, where it promotes research and development in areas including communications, data storage, materials, chemicals, computational sciences, microelectronics, advanced manufacturing and metrology. It drives the development of knowledge-intensive industries through the creation of knowledge and intellectual property, and manages seven research institutes among other facilities.

The A*STAR Joint Council's work takes an interdisciplinary approach to research in the biomedical, physical science, and engineering fields. The Council's mission, according to its website, is "to seed and develop novel scientific discoveries and innovations, leveraging on A*STAR's spectrum of capabilities." It acts as a bridge between the Biomedical Research Council and the Science and Engineering Research Council, enabling researchers to explore new opportunities in science and technology.[27]

Subsidiaries of A*STAR include seven biomedical institutes that do research in support of key industries such as pharmaceuticals, medical technology, and biotechnology. Two of the institutes focus on translating research into clinical applications for medical diagnosis and treatment.[28]

To address the issue of the country's shortage of trained scientists, A*STAR launched programs to fund graduate and post-doctoral studies for Singaporean students. One such program, called the A*STAR Graduate Scholarship Partnership PhD Programme, is aimed at students who wish to pursue a research and development career in science and technology after earning a PhD. The program sends students to selected universities around the world. Currently there are approximately 650 graduate students studying abroad. Returning students join scientists working in the various research institutes. The program requires scholarship recipients to return to Singapore upon completion of their studies for a service commitment of up to three years.[29]

Biomedical Research

A prime example of Singapore's dedication to investing in new medical knowledge is its focus on biomedical research, investigating the causes of and developing treatments for diseases. Mr. Khaw Boon Wan, Singapore's

Minister for Health from 2004 to 2011, said that biomedical science is a pillar of the healthcare system. The country has invested billions of dollars in this area, and Biopolis, a state-of-the-art research and development center is clear evidence of its efforts

So visible, in fact, that Mr. Khaw remarked that as people pay higher taxes, they ask what they are getting in return for this kind of investment. The government's answer is that its medical institutions are focusing on *translational research*, that is, the translation of new knowledge to medical practice that can directly benefit the population. A practical orientation of this kind is much easier for people to accept than a focus on fundamental or pure research.[30]

Biomedical Sciences Initiative

By one estimate, biomedical sciences account for six percent of Singapore's GDP, and manufacturing output in this sector is over S$23 billion.[31] Singapore launched its biomedical sciences initiative in 2000. It was a bold step with the intention of making Singapore the biomedical research and manufacturing hub of Asia. The initiative was designed to invest more than S$3 billion over five years to accelerate development of the program. Incentives were created to bring health-related manufacturers to Singapore. Research institutes focused on genomics, bioinformatics, bioengineering, nanotechnology, molecular and cell biology, and cancer therapies also received support.

- The Biomedical Research Council of A*STAR funds and supports public research initiatives.
- The Economic Development Board's Biomedical Sciences Group promotes private sector manufacturing and research and development activities while Bio*One Capital functions as the biomedical investment arm of Board.
- The Ministry of Health's National Medical Research Council funds and supports public research initiatives, as well as awards medical research fellowships for the development of medical research manpower.

Initiatives that have come out of this approach include establishing research infrastructure, providing venture capital support, and strengthening manpower capabilities.

The initial phase of the initiative focused on developing core public research capabilities in the many areas necessary for advanced research, including bioprocessing chemical synthesis, and genomics, to name just a few. The second phase focused on strengthening the research capabilities for translating laboratory work into clinical applications that would provide advances in the state of healthcare. Consortia initiatives were also launched, in areas such as cancer research, bioimaging, stem cell research, and more. The third phase, which we are currently in, focuses on developing economic opportunities in the biomedical sciences by bringing together research agencies, industries within Singapore, and outside corporations for collaboration and partnerships.[32] This initiative led to the founding in 2005 of the Duke-NUS Graduate Medical School in Singapore. The idea behind this collaboration was to develop a curriculum both to complement and support the research taking place in biomedicine. With an innovative new curriculum, the School looks to produce graduates who are highly-trained medical leaders knowledgeable in clinically-related research. The first class of medical students completed their four years of training in 2011 and has moved on to their residencies. I will have more to say about the medical schools and their role in the healthcare system later in this chapter.

Biopolis

A dramatic symbol of Singapore's commitment to healthcare research and biomedical research in particular, Biopolis, is an impressive complex of seven buildings containing state-of-the-art research laboratories and the latest equipment. The complex was designed to promote and enable collaboration between private corporations and public research institutes and public educational organizations. Biopolis has grown into an international research and development center. The complex attracts scientists, researchers, technicians, and administrators from around the world—currently 2,000 in number.

The buildings provide space and resources for scientific research, and house both public and private laboratories. One key attraction of the site is the close intermingling of public and corporate facilities, affording unique opportunities for cooperation and integration of scientific exploration.

Several government agencies, publicly funded research institutes, and research labs of pharmaceutical and biotechnological companies are found in Biopolis, as well as laboratories for research in neuroscience and immunology.

Included among the many organizations with laboratories and offices in the complex are Singapore's A*STAR biomedical institutes, including the Bioinformatics Institute, Bioprocessing Technology Institute, Genome

Institute of Singapore, Institute of Bioengineering and Nanotechnology, and Institute of Molecular and Cell Biology; Bio*One Capital; laboratories of leading corporations such as the GlaxoSmithKline Centre for Research in Cognitive and Neurodegenerative Disorders; Novartis Institute for Tropical Diseases, which collaborates with A*STAR's Genome Institute in its work; and Fujitsu Laboratories, the first biomedical-focused research facility in Southeast Asia.[33]

Procter & Gamble is creating its Singapore Innovation Centre at Biopolis. The S$250 million premises will house 400 researchers when fully completed in 2013. The Centre will make Procter & Gamble the largest private sector organization at Biopolis and the first to erect its own building. It will undertake development and design of healthcare, beauty and grooming products, as well as new materials research.[34]

Government offices in Biopolis house regulatory agencies involved in drug administration and medical device registration, in order to be available to provide convenient consultation and information, and to address issues in these areas. State-of-the-art equipment and scientific-technological services are available at Biopolis through its Shared Facilities program. It manages and provides core services that researchers need, such as glassware washing and media preparation. Other services available include DNA sequencing, flow cytometry, mass spectrometry, and much more. Singapore's investment in the biomedical industry appears to be paying off. From 2000 to 2007, the manufacturing output of the biomedical industry quadrupled from S$6 billion to over S$24 billion, making it one of the fastest growing sectors in Singapore's economy. The number of workers employed in this sector also increased during that same time period from under 6,000 to almost 12,000. 2010 figures show an output of just under S$23 billion, a workforce numbering almost 14,129 establishments operating in the sector, and a contribution to GDP of 3.5 percent (see Table 7.1).[35]

Achievements in the biopharmaceutical sector include: seven of the world's top pharmaceutical and biotechnology companies investing in 30 manufacturing facilities in Singapore; and the fact that eight of the top ten pharmaceutical companies have their regional headquarters in the country.[36]

With reference to medical technology, Singapore can point to 30 global medical technology companies with commercial-scale manufacturing plants; the country has become one of the world's leading manufacturing sites for research tools and diagnostics instruments; plus, all of the top ten medical technology companies now have their regional headquarters in Singapore.

Table 7.1

STATISTICS BIOMEDICAL INDUSTRY

NUMBER OF ESTABLISHMENTS
2006 2007 2008 2009 2010

VALUE-ADDED ($M)
2006 2007 2008 2009 2010

NUMBER OF WORKERS
2006 2007 2008 2009 2010

VALUE-ADDED PER WORKER ($'000)
2006 2007 2008 2009 2010

TOTAL OUTPUT ($M)
2006 2007 2008 2009 2010

GDP CONTRIBUTION (%)
2006 2007 2008 2009 2010

Industries Size of Total Output	Establishments (No)	Workers (No)	Total Output ($'m)	Value Added ($'m)	Value Added Per Worker ($'000)
Biomedical Engineering	129	13,926	22,759	10,203	732.7
ESTABs with < $1m	59	186	9	-1	-5.5
ESTABs with $1m - < $5m	20	480	57	24	50.1
ESTABs with $5m - < $10m	5	341	40	21	60.4
ESTABs with $10m - < $25m	7	667	120	66	98.3
ESTABs with $25m & above	38	12,252	22,533	10,094	823.9

Source : Economic Development Board,2010 & SPRING Singapore

Private Hospital Healthcare Investments

The private sector is also involved in expanding Singapore's economic foot-print internationally in the healthcare sector. Parkway Pantai Limited, previously headquartered in Singapore but now part of the IHH Healthcare Berhad group, is one of the region's largest integrated private healthcare groups with a network of 17 hospitals and more than 3,000 beds throughout Asia, including Singapore, Malaysia, Brunei, India, China, and Vietnam. From 2013, the Group will have six new hospitals with more than 1,800 additional beds.[37]

In Malaysia, the Group owns and operates 11 hospitals and ancillary healthcare services; in China, nine medical, surgical, and dental centers.

Through 2010, 69 percent of Parkway's billion dollar plus revenue came from Singapore, with 24 percent coming from Southeast Asia and the remainder from North and South Asia.[38]

The Raffles Medical Group also has holdings outside of Singapore, including four medical centers in Hong Kong and Shanghai. It also manages the airport clinics in Singapore's Changi International Airport and Hong Kong's Chek Lap Kok International Airport. Raffles Medical Shanghai is the company's first medical center in China. The company reports that this comprehensive medical center has been growing steadily.

Raffles' revenue in 2011 was S$273 million.[39]

Investing in Healthcare Companies

Singapore's interest in and investment in healthcare extends beyond the borders of the country.

Temasek Holdings

Through Temasek Holdings, an investment company owned by the Government of Singapore (Temasek means *sea town*, the original name of Singapore), the country makes direct investments in companies around the world.[40] Temasek is supported by 12 affiliates and offices in Asia and Latin America, and owns a portfolio valued in the area of S$200 billion, concentrated principally in Asia. Temasek's portfolio covers a broad spectrum of industries: financial services; transportation, logistics and industrials; telecommunications, media and technology; life sciences, consumer and real estate; and energy and resources.

Over the years, Temasek's investments in bioscience and healthcare outside of Singapore have included a joint venture in the pharmaceutical sector with US biotechnology company, Quintiles Transnational Corporation, and Interpharma Asia Pacific, a Hong Kong healthcare company, to commercialize drugs in the Asia Pacific market; an investment in Vical, a US company that researches and develops biopharmaceutical products based on its patented DNA delivery technologies; Matrix Labs (India), Bumrungrad Hospital (Thailand) and Intercell (Austria). In late 2010, it acquired three percent of Max India, a company operating in life insurance, health insurance, healthcare, and clinical research. Temasek has also invested in Shanghai Pharmaceuticals, one of the largest integrated pharmaceutical companies in China.[41]

Temasek operates an extensive philanthropic program. Through its Temasek Trust, it funds, among other organizations, the Singapore Millennium Foundation, which promotes research in mental health, Parkinson's disease, neuromuscular disease, liver cancer, bio-fuel, aging, palliative care, and non-medical bioscience in Singapore; and Temasek Life Sciences Laboratory, a non-profit organization conducting research in molecular biology and genetics.

Other philanthropic endowments and gifts can be seen at its website: http://www.temasek.com.sg/community/temasektrust.[42]

Singapore's Sovereign Wealth Fund

The Government of Singapore Investment Corporation is a fund wholly owned by the government and dedicated to achieving good long-term returns for the government. The fund has offices in nine cities worldwide. Its assets are estimated to be over S$300 billion. The Fund's portfolio is highly diversified across thousands of investments and financial instruments, including public equities, real estate, fixed income, buyout funds, natural resources, and infrastructure.

Over 40 percent of its investments are in the Americas, followed by Europe with almost 30 percent and Asia almost 30 percent. Its interests in emerging economies include investments in China, India, and Latin America.[43]

A System Dedicated to Improving Itself

The Ministry of Health has developed a process to ensure that it looks continually for ways to improve the healthcare system it oversees and the way the Ministry itself and its employees do their jobs—to develop, in a sense, an innovation culture. In 2008, it began using a framework to identify, evaluate, and provide feedback on actions and ideas for improvement. The process involves seeding and generating ideas, bringing relevant parties together in collaboration for testing and experimenting, and implementing the best ideas that survive the vetting process. A few of the initiatives that have arisen in conjunction with the process include establishment of health and wellness programs to enhance the system's public/private partnerships, development of a chronic disease management program, and implementation of the National Mental Health Blueprint. Internal Ministry changes have also taken place including reorganization of the National Medical Research Council.[44]

Looking Abroad for the Best Healthcare Ideas

The quest for the best ideas in high-quality care, efficient processes and procedures, and cost reduction should know no national boundaries. Singapore's healthcare officials know this. While dedicated to improving the system through internal consultation, public feedback, seminars, and more, they also look outward for useful advances taking place in other nations.

Former Health Minister Mr. Khaw Boon Wan shared with me that they do look to India, for example, where pockets of creativity can be found. "For example," he said, "we like the model of eye care, especially cataract care of the Aravind System. They can deliver a cataract surgery at a fully loaded cost of S$100 per patient. Our response has been to hire as many of the Aravind doctors as we can to work here in Singapore." The Ministry of Health told me that in 2011, Singapore brought in about 150 doctors trained in India.

* * *

Chapter 7: KEY POINTS

- Medical education, training, and manpower are provided by two undergraduate medical schools, one postgraduate medical school, a national university, a national science and technology university, and a school of public health
  - ○ The three medical schools each offer a different approach to education and training ranging from the traditional to the radically new
- Singapore is becoming a center for policy research with the establishment of several organizations dedicated to research, thought, and

discussion of issues critical to the future of Singapore, Asia, and the World

- Singapore's Agency for Science, Technology and Research—known as A*STAR—supports key industries, promotes scientific research, develops scientists, and oversees government-sponsored research and development
    - o A*STAR oversees 14 biomedical and physical sciences and engineering research institutes in Singapore
    - o The agency promotes the transition of research into products, services, and new businesses

- Biomedical research initiatives by the government and its agencies seek to make Singapore a key player in the research and development world and also provide benefits to the healthcare system
    - o The main initiative was launched in 2000 with the promise of investing S$3 billion over five years to accelerate the program
    - o Incentives were created to bring health-related manufacturers to Singapore. Research institutes focused on genomics, bioinformatics, bioengineering, nanotechnology, molecular and cell biology, and cancer therapies also received support
    - o Biopolis is a state-of-the-art science and research center designed to promote and enable collaboration between private corporations and public research institutes and public educational organizations

- The private hospital groups in Singapore are expanding internationally, providing Singapore with a broadening economic base in the healthcare sector

- Through Temasek Holdings, the government's investment company, Singapore makes direct investment in individual companies, including many in the healthcare sector. Its philanthropic programs directly benefit healthcare research in Singapore

- The Ministry of Health has put processes in place to identify problems and promote continual improvement in both the administration and delivery of care

CHAPTER 8

Facing the Future

Singapore's Growing Numbers of the Elderly

In many developed countries, the proportion of elderly people in country populations is increasing rapidly. This trend is also true in Singapore, which has for years been experiencing a birth rate substantially below replacement. At the same time that fertility rates have declined, life expectancy has increased—due to the high quality of healthcare and rising standards of living. It is estimated that by 2030, 20 percent of the population will be over 65.[1] The growing proportion of elderly people will have a large impact on the entire society—individuals, families, communities, businesses, and the government.

With its rapidly growing proportion of elderly Singaporeans, managing resources and public expectations in the country has become increasingly complex. The challenge is compounded by the fact that planning for this population shift was generally overlooked during the last 30 years. Now, however, the government is making up for lost time with an aggressive, whole-government response: planning for a future that will require the delivery of more high-quality chronic- and elder-care than ever before and with the goal of increasing expenditures related to GDP by no more than one percent.

Singapore is now embarked on a careful planning and implementation effort involving all government ministries—in effect, a total government effort. It is worth watching and studying what Singapore is doing as it engages all parts of government to accomplish the single goal of preparing for a major increase of elderly in the population. Government ministries and agencies overseeing finance, transportation, housing, social welfare, healthcare, wellness, and more are doing their part. They have even founded a ministerial committee on aging, as I will discuss below.

The surge of seniors is starting right now, as the first of the baby-boomers—the segment of the population born between 1947 and 1964—reach the age of 65.

The generation born in these years has been the main contributor to Singapore's economic expansion and progress over the years. Soon to become the country's seniors, they will be healthier, better educated, more active, and richer than their predecessors.[2]

In fact, a recent study showed that the majority of older Singaporeans report themselves as healthy overall and in a wide range of specific health dimensions.[3] These seniors will not only become influential social and political voices, but they will be an important key consumer group as well. As they age, these elders will contribute to the growth of the "silver industry," fueling the market for goods and services needed or preferred by the elderly, healthcare services included.

The situation Singapore is facing involves new challenges in the delivery of care for these elderly and new challenges for paying for that care. An aging population means more chronic illnesses to treat—diabetes, hypertension, and stroke, for example—more complex medical conditions to consider, more necessary rehabilitation care, a higher demand for transitional support to living at home, convalescence care in nursing homes and aged care facilities, and greater requirements for long-term and end-of-life care.[4]

One study suggests that the burden of care for stroke victims will increase "dramatically" in the years to come due to the growing proportion of elderly people in the population combined with high level of stroke risk factors in Singapore. Currently, stroke is the country's fourth leading cause of death (a rate of 40 per 100,000 in 2006) and among the top ten causes of hospitalization.[5] Another study suggests that there will be an increase in the number and proportion of individuals in the Singapore population with severe dementia. This projection, together with the expected decrease in family size, suggest that many more severe dementia sufferers will be unable to be cared for at home, and new care options are urgently needed.[6] Although it is traditional in Asian societies for families to support their elderly members, the longevity of older people coupled with lower birth rates among the young are making such support increasingly difficult. Simply put, there will be fewer working adults to look after aging family members and to help finance their care. Singapore is preparing its healthcare system for this difficult state of affairs, and in this chapter I will examine the steps being taken to ensure that future needs of the new elderly are met.

At the end of 2012, the government announced a dramatic expansion of eldercare facilities to take place over the next five years. It will spend over S$500 million to build 10 nursing homes, 21 Senior Care Centres, and 45 Senior Activity Centres, with work to be completed by 2016. The additional nursing homes will add over 3,000 beds to Singapore's nursing home capacity, bringing the total number of beds to over 12,000. Minister for Health Gan Kim Yong said in the announcement: "Our goal is to eventually make every neighbourhood a senior friendly neighbourhood, by having aged care facilities that can provide accessible care to seniors living all over the island. Many of these seniors are our pioneers, our parents and our grandparents. We too will age. So this investment in aged care facilities is for Singapore and for our future."[7]

Ministerial Committee on Ageing

Singapore is getting ready for this future. In 2007, a Ministerial Committee on Ageing was established to coordinate aging issues across all government agencies. It is made up of the heads of key government ministries that can contribute to the effort. At its founding, Ministers from the following government departments sat on the Committee: Health; Community Development, Youth and Sports (now restructured as Culture, Community and Youth; and Social and Family Development); National Trades Union Congress; State; Education; Manpower; and the Prime Minister's Office. As I write this book, the committee is headed by Mr. Gan Kim Yong who is also the Minster for Health. The Committee on Ageing has identified three "pillars" supporting a high quality of life for seniors: participation, health, and security. It is working to create an environment throughout Singapore where, as they grow old, individuals can lead lives that are healthy, active, and productive. One focus is on giving families the support they need to take care of their own elderly members, at home, as they age. As Minister Gan has said, "The best medical care in an institution cannot replace a family member's love and support."

The Committee's strategy for seniors is driven by into four initiatives: allowing seniors to stay on the job, drawing salaries and remaining financially independent; enabling the elderly to age in their own communities in a barrier-free environment and with a transportation system that allows them mobility; maintaining a healthcare system that gives seniors access to care for their particular needs at an affordable price; and promoting active aging by encouraging physical and mental well-being and the ability to continue to contribute to society. The Committee on Ageing coordinates the efforts by the various ministries charged with addressing the needs of the elderly and creating an environment for successful aging.[8]

In a 2012 speech, Health Minister Gan Kim Yong outlined the government's priority as continued emphasis on promoting *active* aging through the Wellness Programme, which has already reached 100,000 Singaporeans, and through the Employment Act, which enables individuals to work beyond the statutory retirement age of 62.

Looking ahead to 2020, when it is estimated that the population comprising people above 65 years of age in Singapore will reach 600,000, approximately 85 percent will be functional and healthy—and the government will aggressively push to keep them that way for as long as possible through preventative screening and healthy lifestyle programs. In terms of delivery of healthcare for this population, it plans to at least double the outreach of home-based healthcare services from to eight to 10,000. Social care in the home will also be increased.

There are plans to triple day social and rehabilitative care facilities to over 6,000, as well as to increase the number of Seniors Activity Centres along with the increased staffing and resources needed to run them. Nursing home beds are to be increased by some 70 percent to almost 16,000 by 2020. In order to give the elderly the opportunity to spend their senior years at home with their families, Singapore will expand and enhance new care services, such as stronger transitional care after hospital stays, transitional convalescence facilities to give seniors the rehabilitation they need to return home, in addition to the increase in home-based services.[9]

Agency for Integrated Care

The Agency for Integrated Care (AIC) was established in 2009 by the Ministry of Health to work across care units to improve the standard of care and to effect the integration of primary, intermediate- and long-term care sectors.

Dr. Jason Cheah, CEO of AIC, shared with me that in its efforts to integrate care, his group operates at the patient level, the provider level, and at the system level. They also take direction from what was formerly the Ministry of Community Development, Youth and Sports (now restructured as the Ministry of Culture, Community and Youth; and the Ministry of Social and Family Development). The Agency's main goal is to eventually enable all the various parties at the various levels of care involved with a patient to work together in a more coordinated manner. He is concerned that while the government has made huge investments in the public hospitals, poor people with chronic diseases do not have access to the services they need for ongoing treatment. "When the patients are discharged, the care becomes suboptimal," he said. Transport is also an issue, according to Dr. Cheah. People requiring long-term assistance still have to travel a long distance to get treatment. He sees a very important need for follow-up—community-level care for patients once they are discharged from hospital—so they do not need to return to the hospital.

AIC coordinates and facilitates placing of elderly sick into nursing homes, with community providers, and in day rehabilitation centers. It also handles discharge planning and transition of patients from hospitals to long-term care facilities or to their own homes. In addition, it manages referrals to home care services. According to Dr. Cheah, Agency initiatives over the next two years include better integrated aged care, growing the capacity in home care, and creating new service models as nursing homes are running at full capacity.

Devoted to "meeting the growing healthcare needs of our ageing population," the Agency, according to Dr. Cheah's letter on its website, is "the primary body to advise and guide patients and their families on the use of appropriate healthcare services, and to help you better navigate the healthcare system. We will coordinate, manage and monitor patient referrals to a greater range of Long-Term Care services. AIC will play an active role to support the growth and development of the Primary Care and Long-Term Care sectors, as critical partners in our healthcare system."[10]

With many assistance programs in place to assist the elderly, the Agency for Integrated Care works actively to increase awareness of them and to ensure that the assistance is provided to those in need. It collaborates with grassroots community organizations to conduct outreach, going from door to door to inform the low-income elderly of the different available resources to them.

AIC refers about 6,000 patients to service providers each year of which more than 75 percent are older than 65 and require assistance in activities of daily living such as using the toilet, personal grooming, and feeding, or they may be bed-bound. Over 14,000 patients have been assisted, after hospital discharge to transition to their homes and their community by the Aged Care Transition Initiative.

Among its many other initiatives, the Agency works closely with general practitioners to meet the challenge of the rise of chronic diseases in the populations by bringing together provider networks, developing shared resources, and piloting new models of care. It also administers the Health Manpower Development Programme for Intermediate and Long-Term Care, providing support and funding for education and training programs for workers in elderly and continuing care. It is also piloting enhancement of the

Integrated Home Care Program, bringing new training and new therapies to the fore. According to Dr. Cheah, AIC does "not provide much of the training ourselves. We commission it. We set standards, and mostly in areas of chronic care and mental health."[11]

Center for Enabled Living

Just as the Agency for Integrated Care is an outreach arm of the Ministry of Health, the Center for Enabled Living (CEL) provides an outreach function for the Ministry of Social and Family Development (formerly Community Development, Youth and Sports). The Agency is part of the national care network and is involved in care and support services for the elderly and persons with disabilities. It provides centralized information and referral services, administers eldercare and disability programs, and implements public education programs such as the LivEnabled campaign, which raises awareness of the Centre's work and heightens public knowledge of the various support services available in the community.[12]

The Agency coordinates social care services in support of the frail elderly and persons with disabilities, enabling them to lead independent lives and delaying premature institutionalization. It coordinates and administers schemes and services such as Senior Home Care, Senior Care Centres, Early Intervention Programme for Infants and Children, Caregiver Training Grant, Assistive Technology Fund, Foreign Domestic Worker Grant, and Caregivers Support Programmes. It encourages aging in place, making Singapore a compassionate and inclusive society for the elderly and persons with disabilities, and promotes research and programs toward achieving that goal.[13]

CEL estimates that there are 30,000 elderly Singaporeans above 60 who have difficulties with at least one "activity of daily living," such as washing/bathing, feeding, toileting, transferring, dressing and mobility, and are in need of some form of care support. The number of such elderly is expected to reach 65,000 by 2020. In an effort to bring appropriate levels of care to these individuals, the Centre offers assessment and coordination for enabling, social day care centers, home help services (such as meals delivery and personal hygiene assistance), befriending, neighborhood links for volunteer support, senior activity centers, and sheltered/community homes.

An Integrated Approach to Eldercare

Singapore's healthcare policymakers have realized that effective eldercare requires an integrated approach to infrastructure and have begun forming regional health systems. The intention is to have acute general hospitals linked to community rehabilitation hospitals, supported by collaborative groups of primary care providers, community home care organizations, and rehabilitation centers as partners. To make the patients transition seamlessly from one provider and facility to another, effective coordination between the acute hospitals and their clinical partners in the community is imperative. Singapore's electronic health records system, which I examined in Chapter 7, will support these efforts.

A goal of the integration initiative is to build a strong primary and community care sector that delivers preventive care and comprehensive disease management. With proper care at these lower levels of the system, elderly diabetes patients, for example, can manage their disease without recourse to the acute hospitals. In addition, with good care at the earliest stages of illness, Singaporeans can avoid medical complications and costly hospitalization. Serving a patient with chronic conditions, the system could work as follows.[14]

Patients can take part in an Integrated Screening Programme at a clinic located close to home. The doctor becomes their family physician. Patients are free to see any primary care doctor but might choose to receive care under the Chronic Disease Management Program with a family physician who is trained to provide comprehensive care on an ongoing basis. When visiting the clinic, patients do not have to wait in long lines or expect to be transferred from specialist to specialist due to multiple ailments. The family physician should be able to see to them. Four times a year, the patients and their families, together with other chronic disease patients, attend a Saturday morning class on disease management techniques held by the nurse educator at the community center. The sessions focus on self-administration of medicine, use of medical equipment, and healthy lifestyles and behaviors.

Once a year, patients return to the family physician for a target health assessment which includes a health screening and a review of their medical history along with current health conditions and lifestyle. All the tests are conducted at the clinic, including the more advanced ones requiring sophisticated medical equipment. This is possible because the family physician has grouped with five other general practitioners in the area to jointly acquire that equipment.

Outpatient expenses for consultations, medications and tests are partly covered by Medisave for the Chronic Disease Management Programme. It involves more than 700 general practitioner clinics and groups that provide systematic chronic disease management programs. Patients visiting participating doctors can use their family or their own Medisave (up to 10 accounts) up to S$300 per account per year to pay outpatient bills. Each claim is subject to a deductible of S$30 and a 15 percent co-payment.[15]

Patients' health records are stored on a nationwide Electronic Medical Records are updated in the system whenever they visit a doctor or take a test, and include all of their medical conditions along with the latest medications being taken. If complications arise, the family physician can choose to refer patients to a public hospital. A collaborative team of doctors and other health professionals, led by the family physician, works out a personalized treatment and health progress plan for patients. The team effort is coordinated by a care manager at the hospital who works out the appointments with the collaborative team. The patient is invited to attend the care team meetings to provide feedback on the treatment plan.

Following the hospital visit, patients can join disease management support groups where they can exchange experiences and learn from one another. If a condition is incurable, palliative care, which focuses on preventing and relieving suffering, can be provided at a hospice or at home. The family physician provides counseling on both the clinical and psychological aspects of the situation, and this advice can be complemented by spiritual guidance from the hospice. In case of severe difficulties or complications, the patient can be admitted to a local community hospital and be stabilized there without the need for the costly major hospitals. The family physician can visit patients at the very end of life to ease their pain and help family members navigate the final medical procedures.

Community-Based Care for the Frail Elderly

A new community-based model is underway that allows frail, elderly individuals to receive the high level of continuing care they need while living in their homes and communities, and with their loved ones, instead of being placed in a nursing home. Called the Singapore Programme for Integrated Care for the Elderly, it combines public and private support through rehabilitation centers and day care centers. Personnel in the program are trained to provide quality medical, nursing, and rehabilitation care for these elderly. Elderly patients who are discharged from a hospital can be assessed for suitability for the program and then have the option of enrolling in the program instead of moving permanently to a nursing home. It also provides social workers to support the families in managing their social and emotional difficulties in having frail, elderly family members at home.[16]

The program is not without its challenges. Some people are objecting to the placement of long-term care facilities in their neighborhoods, and the rise of such not-in-my-backyard thinking is giving PAP politicians pause. The issue is one that is currently being negotiated with Singaporeans and tackled on a neighborhood-by-neighborhood basis.[17]

The government will need to mobilize support from within the various neighborhoods to ensure acceptance of these centers. A whole government approach, including targeted communication and engagement by politicians and ministers alike will be necessary to address community concerns and keep the program on track.

Functional Screening Programme

The Health Promotion Board has recently rolled out the Community Functional Screening Programme for seniors aged 60 years and above. Aimed at helping seniors detect early signs of functional decline, the screening focuses on continence, oral health, hearing, vision, and physical function.

Since changes in life such as retirement, loss of loved ones, and worsening health may induce depression, screening is provided for early detection of depression symptoms and enables a medical follow up.

Seniors found to have problems in any of these areas are referred to the proper medical personnel for follow-up testing and treatment.

The physical function test focuses on detecting disability and risks for falls. Seniors with low physical function are referred to family physicians for medical follow ups and are also invited to a 12-week program designed to help them increase their strength and improve their balance.

The screenings are followed up by a nurse counselor on the same day onsite. The results are interpreted and the participants receive guidance on the appropriate medical follow up and healthy lifestyle practices.

Private Initiatives in Support of the Elderly

Numerous non-governmental organizations in Singapore provide funding, support, and a range of services for the elderly. One very prominent group is the Tsao Foundation, and it will be instructive to take a closer look at its initiatives.

The Tsao Foundation

The Tsao Foundation is a not-for-profit organization dedicated to enhancing the quality of life for older people. It pioneers new approaches to care, provides duplicable models of health services, and attempts to fill in the gaps in eldercare services.

One of the Foundation's missions is to provide services that will enable elderly persons to remain in their own homes and communities as long as possible and avoid premature placement in nursing homes. The Tsao Foundation acts through its Hua Mei Community Health Services, a comprehensive, community-based primary healthcare system consisting of a mobile clinic, an outpatient primary geriatric care facility, a pain management center, and a care management center for those with complex medical problems, financial needs, and little social support.

The Foundation also manages training programs with the aim of fostering higher standards of eldercare in Singapore. The programs provide training for long-term care and health professionals, volunteers and family caregivers on different topics: eldercare, dementia care, health promotion, and the psycho-emotional dimensions of aging.[18] The Foundation has also developed partnerships with other care organizations in the furtherance of its mission. Its training academy, for example, works with the National Council of Social Services and the Social Service Training Institute, providing professional courses and training manuals. It also offers pre-retirement training programs to corporations, focusing on physical, emotional, and financial well-being preparing employees for retirement and successful aging. The Tsao Foundation also contributes to eldercare policy planning and development by engaging policymakers in dialogue, providing research, and participating in government committee work.

Helping the Elderly Pay for Care

I have already discussed the benefits and uses of the Central Provident Fund and its healthcare components, Medisave, MediShield, and Medifund—the 3Ms of the Singapore system. They are an important factor in helping Singaporeans pay their medical and other healthcare bills. With people living longer, the possibility, especially among the elderly, of running out of money to pay for care becomes very real. Medifund, the endowment fund to help needy citizens, and Medifund Silver, which sets aside a specific amount of money in Medifund for assisting individuals over 65, are especially relevant to the present discussion.

In Chapter 3, I discussed at length the role of Medifund. I note again here, though, that seniors who have no or very little money in their Medisave accounts are given priority for Medifund payouts.[19] In addition, Medifund Silver, launched in November 2007, another endowment fund created by the government, is specially targeted at helping the elderly poor. Further, Medifund has been extended to cover patients in approved private nursing homes.

I see these actions as more evidence of the government's ongoing commitment to fine tune the system as conditions change—in these instances, of course, responding to the needs of the growing numbers of the elderly in Singapore.

Annuity Programs

The latest addition to initiatives to aid the elderly is an annuity program called CPF LIFE (Central Provident Fund—Lifelong Income For the Elderly). Its goal is to provide lifelong income to the elderly and it involves transferring part of CPF retirement savings into an annuity starting at age 55. The annuity begins working at age 62 to 65, depending on when the individual was born, and provides a steady monthly stream of income for life. Individuals can sign up for CPF LIFE between the ages of 55 and 80.

Starting with members who will turn 55 in 2013, those with at least S$40,000 in their Retirement Account will be automatically included in the program, while those with lower balances may still opt in. Upon joining CPF LIFE, depending on age, gender, and the plan selected, a certain percentage of Retirement Account savings will be transferred to the CPF LIFE account as premium for the annuity.[20]

There are several different plans in the program that adjust the level of payout against the amount of money left for beneficiaries upon the death of the individual. The higher the payout, the lower the balance left over for a bequest. For example, a 55-year-old woman joining the program would receive an amount from just over S$700 to something under S$900 monthly depending on the plan she chooses. A 55-year-old man choosing the plan with the highest monthly payout would be using his entire retirement savings to purchase the annuity.[21]

Initiatives in the Healthcare Budget

At this time of writing, Singapore's 2012 budget is in effect. The budget contains numerous provisions for helping the elderly afford their care, again illustrating the government's willingness to tweak the system when conditions change or new challenges arise. Older workers aged 50 years and above receive a bump—up to 2.5 percent—in their employers' Central Provident Fund contributions; at the same time, to help companies with the increased costs, those who hire older workers will receive a new wage subsidy of eight percent. Such measures enable individuals, now living and staying healthy longer, to continue earning salaries well beyond the retirement years established in the past.

There are increased subsidies for nursing home care, day care, rehabilitation, and home-based care. Two-thirds of households will qualify for the increases. Subsidized patients at community hospitals, nursing homes, or using home care services will no longer have to pay the seven percent tax on goods and services formerly applied to their bills.

The government seems especially interested in helping the elderly remain in their homes and with their families: families taking care of an elderly parent at home could see their monthly cost of care go down from S$1,400 to S$700 per month, according to government estimates. There is even a S$120 grant to hire a maid to help with care of a senior. Plus we are seeing a new subsidy to install elderly-friendly features in the home.[22]

Infrastructure Improvements

The 2012 budget provides funds and establishes goals for 1,900 more beds in the general hospitals by 2020 (a 30 percent increase); four new community hospitals by 2020 adding 1,800 new beds; new intermediate- and long-term care facilities, expansion of nursing home capacities along with new nursing homes. In addition, long-term care facilities will be repositioned near major residential towers so patients can be close to their families. Along with various voucher plans, utility rebates, and Medisave top ups, the government is attempting to make sure the Singapore safety net keeps up with the times and allows the elderly and the poor to receive the aid they need.

Staffing Up for Eldercare

More doctors, nurses, and other healthcare professionals will be needed to take care of the elderly and to staff the infrastructure expansion antici-pated in the budget, and funds are being allocated for that purpose. The medical needs of the elderly require the support of many different healthcare professionals. In the past, it was thought that the doctor, nurse, physiotherapist, occupational therapist, and medical social worker formed the necessary team to care for seniors. The Singapore healthcare system recognizes through its policies and initiatives the need for additional allied health professionals, including speech therapists, dietitians, case managers, psychologists, dentists, optometrists and podiatrists.

Doctors required for high-quality eldercare include specialists in the acute hospitals and family physicians for long-term care. In intermediate care, both types of physicians play a role. Doctors who become geriatricians are trained in biomedical and social aspects of aging, including the sociology of aging, quality of life, healthcare ethics, elderly mistreatment, and the impact of the caregiver on the quality of care.[23]

The increasing importance of geriatric nursing is being recognized, and training advancements have been made with the establishment of an Advanced Diploma in Gerontological Nursing offered at Nanyang Polytechnic. The Singapore Nurses Association has stated as a mission the goal of bringing Gerontological Nursing to the forefront as a specialist field.[24] Increasing numbers of other personnel who serve the elderly, such as physiotherapists, occupational therapists, and speech therapists, are needed and are being recruited through a Ministry of Health pilot employment initiative mentioned in Chapter 6. With this program, these professionals would be recruited centrally to be deployed at intermediate and long-term care institutes and hospitals.[25]

Additionally, the government is reaching out to the private practitioners who overwhelmingly provide primary healthcare services in Singapore and is offering them greater roles in providing preventive and monitoring services to the elderly. Many of such clinics are located close to HDB flats where over 80 percent of the Singapore population resides.[26] Through programs such as the Community Health Assist Scheme (examined in Chapter 6), these private practitioners can contribute a great deal to eldercare, keeping the senior population healthier, bringing costs down, and relieving the strain on acute hospitals from unnecessary hospitalizations.

Even the elderly are being trained to take care of the elderly. One example is the Senior Health Ambassador Programme administered by the Health Promotion Board. People aged 40 and above are invited to join, participate in workshops, exercise classes and health cooking demonstrations. They are then asked to take their knowledge and enthusiasm for healthy living into their communities and inspire others to attain a healthy lifestyle. As the HPB states on its website, "Let us help you lead the way in providing health advice to your family and friends to achieve a healthier and happier life."[27]

*　　* *

Chapter 8: KEY POINTS

- Singapore's birth rate is substantially lower than the replacement rate
  - By 2030, 20 percent of the population will be over 65
  - The country is preparing now for the impact these demographics will have on society

- The Ministerial Committee on Ageing coordinates aging issues across all government agencies
  - At its founding, Ministers from the following government departments sat on the Committee: Health; Community Development, Youth and Sports (now restructured as Culture, Community and Youth; and Social and Family Development); National Trades Union Congress; State; Education; Manpower; and the Prime Minister's Office
  - The four key initiatives are: allow seniors to stay on the job longer and remain financially independent; provide barrier-free environments and transportation for the elderly; give seniors access to care for their particular needs at an affordable price; promote active aging

- The Agency for Integrated Care works across care units to improve the standard of care and to effect the integration of primary, intermediate- and long-term care sectors—all areas of increasing importance as the elderly population swells

- The healthcare system is transforming itself into regional systems. Acute general hospitals to be linked to community rehabilitation hospitals, supported by groups of primary care providers, community home care organizations, and rehabilitation centers as partners

- Community-based care for the frail elderly is another initiative and an alternative to nursing homes
  - Allows the frail elderly to receive the continuing care they need while living in their homes and communities, and with their loved ones, instead of in a nursing home

- Private initiatives in support of the elderly play an important role in eldercare—one important example is The Tsao Foundation
  - The Foundation pioneers new approaches to care, provides duplicable models of health services, and attempts to fill in the gaps in eldercare services

- Medifund, the endowment fund to help needy citizens, and Medifund Silver, which sets aside a specific amount of money in Medifund for assisting individuals over 65 help the elderly pay for their care

    o   Annuity programs are being added to the Central Provident Fund to help provide older Singaporeans a steady monthly stream of income for life

    o   The 2012 Singapore budget provides numerous provisions for helping the elderly afford their care, illustrating the government's willingness to tweak the system when conditions change or new challenges arise

Appendix

Q&A with the Ministry of Health, Singapore

In addition to interviews and public sources of data consulted, I put a number of questions to Singapore's Ministry of Health in writing. This appendix includes a selection of the questions and written responses I received. They are reproduced here to give a more direct sense of the Ministry's approach to particular issues, or because they provide useful supplementary detail.

1. *In my discussions of the Singapore healthcare system, many knowledgeable people comment that the success of the system is due to the country's small size and cannot be replicated on a larger scale. How do you respond to this comment?*

    Singapore's healthcare system has evolved to meet the needs of its people, taking into account demographic, epidemiological, socio-economic and historical factors. Our small size and highly urbanized environment have made it easier to roll out public health programs such as clean water, good sanitation, and immunization programs; and has also made it easy for all Singaporeans to have access to good-quality healthcare services at all levels. Beyond these, other key success factors of Singapore's healthcare system include efficient processes, sound and sustainable financing systems, personal ownership of health, among others. Arguably, these are not contingent on a country's size, but rather its cultural context and governance system.

2. *In my conversations with officials in Singapore, they often mention that, although the healthcare system may not be applicable to a large country, it may be appropriate for large cities. Do you agree with this assertion?*

    Singapore's healthcare system has developed within the context of a city-state environment, where there is higher population density, road networks, and proximity to healthcare infrastructure. The applicability of the Singapore model to other cities would depend on their specific historical, economic and social context, cultural norms and beliefs, and governance systems.

3.   *A common reaction to my discussions of the Singapore healthcare system is to dismiss its success because Singapore is a "dictatorship," or because it has such an unusual form of government that the healthcare system cannot be replicated elsewhere. How do you respond to these reactions?*

Many key elements of our healthcare system have their origins in our years as a British colony, including the system of medical and nursing education, the delivery and organisation of care where care was provided free at the point of delivery, and even the Central Provident Fund introduced by the British in 1953 to help individuals save for their own retirement needs from which a portion was carved out later to form the medical savings account. Since then, Singapore's healthcare system has evolved. The strong political leadership certainly helped shape the healthcare system. But, there were other historical, institutional, economic, and social factors which also played a part.

For example, whilst Singapore had inherited a UK-style NHS system from the British upon independence, the Singapore government grew concerned about the possibilities of unrestrained growth in demand and healthcare costs. Thus, co-payments were slowly introduced and the healthcare system gradually evolved to a market-based hybrid-funded model premised on personal responsibility with government support.

Several key conditions in Singapore facilitated this evolution. First, we had a young and healthy population, with a high savings rate. Second, the concept of mandatory retirement savings had been introduced early, paving the way for public acceptance of the need to save for post-retirement costs. Third, there was a general cultural alignment on the philosophy that each person was responsible for looking after his own health and that of his family. These key factors allowed the government to build on the CPF Board to institute mandatory health savings accounts under the overall retirement savings framework. Thereafter, insurance through MediShield and the Medifund safety net were introduced over time to strengthen the healthcare financing framework for Singaporeans.

4.   *What are the data on the Medisave savings of the self-employed? Do they save proportionally the same amount of money as those who are employed by*

businesses? If not, is the lack of savings posing a strain on the self-employed or on the system?

All self-employed persons earning more than S$6,000 in annual net trade income are required to contribute to Medisave. Their Medisave contribution rates are broadly in line with that for employees, and are phased in according to income. Those with net trade income of more than S$18,000 a year contribute the full rates, currently ranging from 7% to 9%* depending on age. Those with net trade income above S$6,000 but below S$12,000 contribute one-third of the full rates. Although self-employed persons with net trade income of S$6,000 or below are not required to contribute Medisave, they are encouraged to do so voluntarily to build up their healthcare savings.

Unlike employees whose Medisave contributions are automatically deducted from their salary by the employer and credited to their Medisave accounts, self-employed persons have to make the contributions themselves and hence the Medisave compliance rate is lower. As at May 2012, 85% of all registered self-employed persons complied with their Medisave contribution requirements. Government measures to raise compliance include both education and enforcement efforts.

Self-employed persons are eligible to receive Workfare Income Supplement (WIS) benefits if they meet the qualifying criteria and contribute to Medisave. Their WIS benefits will be paid into their Medisave accounts, and this will add further to their healthcare adequacy.

5.   *With more private practitioners providing primary care through the Community Health Assist Scheme, how will you monitor and measure the quality of care?*

Patients on the Community Health Assist Scheme (CHAS) with chronic conditions are required to enroll in the Chronic Disease Management Programme (CDMP). CDMP seeks to ensure good chronic disease management through the use of evidence-based structured clinical treatment protocols. Apart from following the clinical protocol, providers on the CDMP (including private practitioners) are required to submit their patient's clinical indicators, e.g. HbA1c score for Diabetics, to the Ministry of Health. The results

---

* With effect from 1 Jan. 2013, the Medisave contribution rates for self-employed persons aged 50 and above will be raised from 9.0% to 9.5%. With this change, the range for the full Medisave contribution rates will be 7.0% to 9.5%.

of the indicators are monitored and published by MOH to encourage GPs to improve overall clinical standards.

6. *Regarding private nursing home care eligible for subsidy—how do you monitor and measure the quality of care?*

MOH has been actively coordinating, integrating and improving services more effectively so that our seniors can be cared for better. It expects these measures to be a joint responsibility—the government's role is to provide a robust regulatory and quality framework for aged care, while commercial and Voluntary Welfare Organization (VWO) service providers are expected to constantly improve care delivery and put in place a dynamic structure within their institutions to ensure that care professionals uphold the standards of care required.

MOH started its first portable subsidy scheme for nursing home beds in 2008 to buy subsidized beds from private nursing homes. This is done through a Request for Proposal (RFP) exercise which is effective over a two-year term. Proposals from the private nursing homes are assessed based on operators' compliance to regulatory standards and service-related requirements.

In 2012, various additional measures were introduced to nursing home residents and their caregivers, such as the Nursing Home Visitors' Programme, to provide feedback on care services. The government is also reviewing existing standards and guidelines for aged care services with participation from internal and external stake-holders including clinicians, geriatricians, pharmacists, and nursing home service providers.

7. *Please describe how the quality of care is monitored in the private hospitals.*

The Singapore Healthcare System relies on a multi-pronged approach to monitor the quality of care in the private sector.

First, ensuring that care is of high quality is the responsibility of healthcare professionals. This is regardless of whether care is provided in the public or private sector, or whether in primary care, nursing homes, or hospitals. Accordingly, monitoring the quality of care starts by monitoring the training and practice of healthcare professionals. The Singapore Medical Council and the Specialist Accreditation Board in the Ministry of Health ensure that there is high quality of training for medical doctors in Singapore, and that only suitably trained doctors are licensed to practice in Singapore. Similar agencies/boards exist for other healthcare professionals. These agencies/boards also monitor complaints against any healthcare professionals.

Second, through the National Quality Assurance Framework (NQAF), MOH monitors the compliance of doctors in both public and private sectors to self-regulatory and learning requirements. The aim of the NQAF is to ensure active learning amongst peers, professional norming to high standards of care, as well as to prevent recurrence of harm from medical adverse events. Monitoring compliance to NQAF requirements provides the Ministry with valuable information on the hospitals' ability to ensure high professional standards, to prevent ongoing harm, and to continuously improve.

Third, a set of evidence and best practice based clinical standards and indicators have been developed for public and private hospitals. This is part of the overall national performance measurement framework, comprising the national-level National Health System Scorecard, which is then cascaded to setting- and provider/specialty-level scorecards.

The Scorecards leverage extensively on the indicators developed under the OECD Healthcare Quality Indicator (HCQI) Project. This allows MOH to benchmark Singapore's performance with OECD countries on a "like-for-like" basis, enabling it to identify areas where it is doing well, and where improvements are needed to close quality gaps. For example, the OECD HCQI's indicators on hospitalizations for ambulatory care sensitive conditions enabled the Ministry to monitor the national Chronic Disease Management Programme (which covered conditions such as diabetes, hypertension, asthma, etc.) to successfully reduce hospitalizations.

Finally, a traditional licensing based regulatory approach underpins all of the above. MOH conducts licensing audits of all hospitals, clinics, and nursing homes in Singapore, whether in the private or public sector. Patient complaints to the Ministry are also tracked and investigated.

Notes

Chapter 1

1. National University of Singapore Initiative to Improve Health in Asia (NIHA) Forum in Singapore in 2010.
2. Lee Kuan Yew, *From Third World to First: The Singapore Story 1965–2000* (New York: HarperCollins Publishers, 2000).
3. Yong Nyuk Lin, address at a World Health Organization seminar, Singapore, 1967. Cited in Lim Meng-Kin, "Health Care Systems in Transition II. Singapore, Part I. An Overview of Health Care Systems in Singapore," *Journal of Public Health Medicine* 20, 1 (1998): 16–22. Available at http://jpubhealth. oxfordjournals.org/content/20/1/16.full.pdf
4. Singapore Department of Statistics, "Time Series on GDP at 2005 Market Prices and Real Economic Growth." Available at http://www.singstat.gov. sg/stats/themes/economy/hist/gdp1.html.
5. Lee, *From Third World to First*, p. 95.
6. Ibid., p. 96
7. *Our Quality Journey: Singapore's Healthcare Milestones* (Singapore: Ministry of Health, 2010).
8. Speech by Lee Kuan Yew at the Imperial College Commemoration Eve Dinner. Available at http://www3.imperial.ac.uk/newsandeventspggrp/imperial college/alumni/pastukevents/newssummary/news_26-2-2007-14-0-12.
9. Lim, "Health Care Systems in Transition II."
10. *Our Quality Journey.*
11. Lim, "Health Care Systems in Transition II."
12. Ibid.
13. Available at http://www.nhg.com.sg/nhg_01_pressRelease2003_5july. asp?pr=2003.
14. http://www.asiaone.com/Health/News/Story/A1Story20090818-161867.html; http://www.healthxchange.com.sg/News/Pages/Easier-to-bring-in-foreign-trained-doctors.aspx.
15. Lim, "Health Care Systems in Transition II."
16. Housing and Development Board Infoweb. Available at http://www.hdb. gov.sg/fi10/fi10320p.nsf/w/AboutUsHDBHistory?OpenDocument. See also Barrington Kaye 1961.

17. HDB InfoWEB, HDB History. Available at http://www.hdb.gov.sg/fi10/fi10320p.nsf/w/AboutUsHDBHistory?OpenDocument [accessed 28 Oct. 2011].

18. Lim, "Health Care Systems in Transition II."

19. K.H. Phua, *Social Health Insurance: Selected Case Studies from Asia and the Pacific*, WHO South East Asia Region, New Delhi and Western Pacific Region, Manila, 2005; C.C. Hin, "Planning for the Future—The National Health Plan," *Singapore Medical Journal* 28, 3 (1987): 210–3.

20. Lim, "Health Care Systems in Transition II."

21. C.M. Toh, S.K. Chew, and C.C. Tan, "Prevention and Control of Non-Communicable Diseases in Singapore: A Review of National Health Promotion Programmes," *Singapore Med Journal* 43, 7 (2002) 333–9.

22. M. Ramesh, "Autonomy and Control in Public Hospital Reforms in Singapore," *The Americal Review of Public Administration* 38, 1 (2008): 18.

23. Ministry of Health, *Affordable Health Care—A White Paper* (Singapore: Singapore National Printers for the Ministry of Health, 1993), p. 70.

24. S.C. Emmanuel, S.L. Lam et al., "A Countrywide Approach to the Control of Non-Communicable Diseases—The Singapore Experience," *Ann Acad Med* 31, 4 (2002): 474–8.

25. Y.P. Lim, "Sharing Singapore's Experience in Dietetic Practice and School Nutrition Programmes," *Asia Pac J Clin Nutr.* 17, Supp 1 (2008): 361–4.

26. Ministry of Health, *Affordable Health Care—A White Paper*, p. 70.

27. Available at http://www.channelnewsasia.com/stories/singaporelocalnews/view/327682/1/.html.

Chapter 2

1. Lee Kuan Yew, *From Third World to First: The Singapore Story 1965–2000* (New York: HarperCollins Publishers, 2000), p. 58.

2. WHO National Health Accounts.

3. F. Liew, L.W. Ang et al., "Evaluation on the Effectiveness of the National Childhood Immunisation Programme in Singapore, 1982–2007," *Ann Acad Med Singapore* 39, 7 (2010): 532–10.

4. Singapore Cancer Registry, *Cancer Survival in Singapore 1968–2007* (Singapore: Health Promotion Board, 2011).

5. R. Sankaranarayanan, R. Swaminathan et al., "Cancer Survival in Africa, Asia, and Central America: A Population-Based Study," *Lancet Oncology* 11, 2 (2010): 165–73.

6. The Organisation for Economic Co-operation and Development (OECD), *Health at a Glance: Asia/Pacific 2010* (Paris: OECD, 2010).

7. OECD, *Health at a Glance 2009: OECD Indicators* (Paris: OECD 2009), p. 200.

8. http://www.moh.gov.sg/content/moh_web/home/statistics/Health_Facts_Singapore/Disease_Burden.html.

9. Ministry of Health, "Patient Satisfaction Survey 2010," 2010. Available at http://www.moh.gov.sg/mohcorp/pressreleases.aspx?id=25992 [accessed 10 Oct. 2011].

10. World Health Organization, *The World Health Report 2000 Health Systems: Improving Performance* (Geneva: WHO, 2000).

11. Jennifer B. Boyd; Mary H. McGrath, and John Maa, "Emerging Trends in the Outsourcing of Medical and Surgical Care," *JAMA Surgery* 146, 1 (2011): 107–12.

Chapter 3

1. G. T. Boon, "Provident Fund Gets a Big Welcome," *The Singapore Free Press*, 1 Dec. 1953, p. 12. Available at http://newspapers.nl.sg/Digitised/Article/freepress19531201.2.55.aspx.

2. NIHA Forum: Singapore, Nov. 2010. Khaw Boon Wan, "The Art and Science of Health Care Policy."

3. http://www.singaporemedicalguide.com/hospital-ward-classes/.

4. "Medisave Scheme" *CPF Trends*, Mar. 2011. Available at http://mycpf.cpf.gov.sg/NR/rdonlyres/B9577B11-693D-4E34-A83D-123E1F7731D4/0/MedisaveScheme_Trends_March2011.pdf [10 Dec. 2011]; http://ask-us.cpf.gov.sg/exploreMQA.asp?projectid=1734594&category=23139&strPrint=22994.

5. Ministry of Health, "Withdrawal Limits. Costs and Financing: Schemes & Subsidies, Medisave." Available at http://www.moh.gov.sg/content/moh_web/home/costs_and_financing/schemes_subsidies/medisave.html [accessed 10 Nov. 2011].

6. http://www.hpb.gov.sg/programmes/article.aspx?id=3324; http://www.moh.gov.sg/content/moh_web/home/pressRoom/pressRoomItemRelease/2011/extending_medisaveforscreeningmammogramsandcolonoscopies.html.

7. S. Khalik, "Health Subsidies Extended to 710,000," *Straits Times*, 16 Aug. 2011, p. 2.

8. http://www.singstat.gov.sg/stats/keyind.html#birth; http://www.indexmundi.com/singapore/total_fertility_rate.html.

9. http://202.157.171.46/whitepaper/downloads/population-white-paper.pdf

10. Central Provident Fund, "My CPF—Having Children: Providing for Your Precious Ones. Life Events: Having Children: Immediate Concerns 2011." Available at http://mycpf.cpf.gov.sg/CPF/my-cpf/have-child/HC2.htm [accessed 1 Dec. 2011]. Ministry of Health, "Marriage and Parenthood Schemes. Costs and Financing: Schemes and Subsidies 2011." Available at http://www.moh.gov.sg/content/moh_web/home/costs_and_financing/schemes_subsidies/Marriage_and_Parenthood_Schemes.html [accessed 15 Nov. 2011].

11. http://www.channelnewsasia.com/stories/singaporelocalnews/view/1249234/1/.html.

12. https://www.babybonus.gov.sg/bbss/html/index.html.
13. Ministry of Health, "Use of Medisave for Pneumococcal Vaccination," 2009. Available at http://www.moh.gov.sg/content/moh_web/home/pressRoom/pressRoomItemRelease/2009/use_of_medisave_for_pneumococcal_vaccination.html [accessed 7 Dec. 2011]. Ministry of Health, "Hepatitis B Immunisation Programme," 2001. Available at https://http://www.moh.gov.sg/content/moh_web/home/pressRoom/pressRoomItemRelease/2001/hepatitis_B_immunisation_programme.html [accessed 10 Nov. 2011]. National Healthcare Group Polyclinics, "Child Health Services: Immunisation and Child Development. National Healthcare Group Polyclinics: Our Services 2011." Available at http://www.nhgp.com.sg/ourservices.aspx?id=5000000013 [accessed 10 Nov. 2011]. S. Khalik, "Cervical Cancer Jabs Covered by Medisave," *Straits Times*, 5 Oct. 2010. Ministry of Health, "Medisave 400 Scheme. FAQs: Policies." Available at http://www.pqms.moh.gov.sg/apps/fcd_faqmain.aspx?qst=2fN7e274RAp%2BbUzLdEL%2FmJu3ZDKARR3p5Nl92FNtJiewnENBNFEIiRHmMoeVHrwwzGA%2BwFOVoSHTBVPEq9DECk2raoDSEH38mKUHHqhk8DNKUIN0LEZB7u5R8QnS8ViteA1ZHO8%2FJ69cMiJ3pMFKfSbDdcjb9lI1j7OsjaVpXP7wy%2F5C36hQHIXBtwt%2BNFxi9CoSAkmphWY%3D [accessed 10 Nov. 2011].
14. "Grow and Share' Package Overview," 2011. Available at http://www.growandshare.gov.sg/Overview.htm [accessed 4 Dec. 2011].
15. Workfare Income Supplement Scheme: http://mycpf.cpf.gov.sg/Members/Gen-info/WIS/WIS_Scheme.htm; GST Voucher Scheme: http://gstvoucher.gov.sg/.
16. J.F. Lim and V.D. Joshi, "Public Perceptions of Healthcare in Singapore," *Ann Acad Med Singapore* 37, 2 (2008): 91–5.
17. M.D. Barr, "Medical Savings Accounts in Singapore: A Critical Inquiry," *J Health Polit Policy Law* 26, 4 (2001): 709–26.
18. W. Dong, "Can Health Care Financing Policy be Emulated? The Singaporean Medical Savings Accounts Model and Its Shanghai Replica," *J Public Health* 28, 3(2006): 209–14.
19. http://mycpf.cpf.gov.sg/NR/rdonlyres/78E52772-ED48-4477-9167-28A31DE2566B/0/CPFTrends_Medishield.pdf.
20. http://www.channelnewsasia.com/stories/singaporelocalnews/view/1183628/1/.html.
21. General Information on MediShield Scheme. Available at http://ask-us.cpf.gov.sg/Home/Hybrid/themes/CPF/Uploads/Healthcare/General Information on MSH.pdf [accessed 2 Jan. 2012].
22. Ministry of Health, "How MediShield Works." Available at http://www.moh.gov.sg/content/moh_web/home/costs_and_financing/schemes_subsidies/MediShield/How_MediShield_Works.html]; http://ask-us.cpf.gov.sg/Home/Hybrid/themes/CPF/Uploads/Healthcare/General%20Information%20on%20MSH.pdf.
23. Ministry of Health, "10 Top Common Myths of Singapore Health Care. Press Room: Highlights: 2011," 2011. Available at http://www.moh.gov.sg/content/

moh_web/home/pressRoom/highlights/2011/10_top_common_myths_of_
singapore_health_care.html [accessed 10 Dec. 2011].

24. Ministry of Health personal communication, 2012

25. CPF, "Private Medical Insurance Scheme (PMIS). Meeting Your Healthcare
     Needs." Available at http://ask-us.cpf.gov.sg/explorefaq.asp?category=23069
     [accessed 2 Jan. 2012].

26. http://www.income.com.sg/insurance/i-Medicare/index.asp.

27. Ministry of Health, "ElderShield. Home: Costs and Financing: Schemes and
     Subsidies." Available at https://http://www.moh.gov.sg/content/moh_web/
     home/costs_and_financing/schemes_subsidies/ElderShield.html [accessed 10
     Jan. 2012].

28. http://ask-us.cpf.gov.sg/exploreMQA.asp?projectid=1734594&category=2307
     1&strpage=0&strPrint=#4185193.

29. Tan Weizhen, "ElderShield Scheme Review Will Not Be Rushed," *TODAY*,
     30 Apr. 2012.

30. https://www.moh.gov.sg/content/moh_web/home/costs_and_financing/
     schemes_subsidies/ElderShield/ElderShield_Supplements.html.

31. http://www.moh.gov.sg/content/moh_web/home/costs_and_financing/
     schemes_subsidies/Medifund.html.

32. Singapore Budget 2011, "Benefits for Households. Singapore Budget: Key
     Budget Initiatives." Available at http://www.mof.gov.sg/budget_2011/key_
     initiatives/families.html [accessed 2 Dec. 2012].

33. M. Singh, "Health and Health Policy in Singapore," *ASEAN Economic Bulletin*
     16, 3 (1999): 330–43.

34. Ministry of Health, "Medifund. Home: Costs and Financing: Schemes and
     Subsidies." Available at http://www.moh.gov.sg/content/moh_web/home/
     costs_and_financing/schemes_subsidies/Medifund.html [accessed 15 Jan.
     2012].

35. FAQ from the government.

Chapter 4

1. National Coalition on Health Care, "Health Care Spending as Percentage
    of GDP Reaches All-Time High," 12 Sept. 2011. Available at http://nchc.
    org/node/1171.

2. M.K. Lim, "Transforming Singapore Health Care: Public–Private Partnership,"
    Ann Acad Med Singapore 34, 7 (2005): 461–7.

3. R. Gauld, N. Ikegami et al., "Advanced Asia's Health Systems in Comparison,"
    Health Policy 79, 2–3 (2006): 325–36.

4. Sam Ro, "Revealed: The Cost of Health Insurance around the World," *Business
    Insider*, 26 Apr. 2012. Available at http://www.businessinsider.com/cost-of-
    health-insurance-around-the-world-2012-4#ixzz1zZizuLFo.

5. Salma Khalik, "Medisave Can be Used in 12 M'sian Hospitals," *Straits Times*,
    15 Feb. 2010. Available at http://www.asiaone.com/Health/News/Story/
    A1Story20100216-198974.html.

6. NIHA Forum: Singapore, Nov. 2010. Khaw Boon Wan, "The Art and Science of Health Care Policy."

7. Jonas Schreyögg and Lim Meng Kin, "Health-Care Reforms in Singapore—Twenty Years of Medical Savings Accounts," *CESifo DICE Report*, Ifo Institute for Economic Research at the University of Munich 2, 3 (Oct. 2004): 55–60; Phua Kai Hong, "Attacking Hospital Performance on Two Fronts: Network Corporatization and Financing Reforms in Singapore," in *Innovations in the Delivery of Health Services: The Corporatization of Public Hospitals*, ed. A.S. Preker and A. Harding (Washington, DC: World Bank, 2003), pp. 7–9.

8. Phua, "Attacking Hospital Performance on Two Fronts," in *Innovations in Health Service Delivery: The Corporatization of Public Hospitals*, Volume 434, ed. Alexander S. Preker and April Harding (Washington, DC: World Bank, 2003), p. 468. Available at http://books.google.com/books?id=iFIVuwFa7GE C&pg=PA468&lpg=PA468&dq=revenue+caps+at+Singapore+public+hospital s&source=bl&ots=v5l7Vmi4oF&sig=ZTg_4Z8spwAxkG1xaafMZYpA_KI& hl=en&sa=X&ei=IizOT8jwNIX76gGjqayxDA&ved=0CHEQ6AEwBg#v=on epage&q=revenue%20caps%20&f=false.

9. Quoted in Niko Karvounis, "Health Care in Singapore," in *Taking Note: A Century Foundation Group Blog*. Available at http://takingnote.tcf.org/2008/07/health-care-in.html.

10. http://www.geraldtan.com/premed/Doctor_salaries.html.

11. B. Knight, "No-Fault Compensation and Performance Review," *Ann Acad Med Singapore* 22, 1 (1993): 61–4.

12. W.O. Poon, "Malpractice and Negligence in the Medical Professions," *Singapore Medical Journal* 24, 3 (1983).

13. United States Agency for International Development, "Medical Malpractice Law 'Best Practices' for Jordan," 21 Aug. 2007.

14. Margaret Fordham, "The Law of Negligence." Available at http://www.singaporelaw.sg/content/Negligence.html.

15. http://www.patient-help.com/.

16. http://www.medicalprotection.org/singapore/aboutmps/discretion.

17. http://www.medicalprotection.org/Default.aspx?DN=31cbb51f-e7d4-4feb-9769-ea30cb040ab5.

18. Y.C. Chee, "Do No Harm: Do Thyself No Harm, 2005 SMA Lecture," *Singapore Med J* 46, 12 (2005): 667.

19. Ibid.

20. http://pss.org.sg.

21. Jeremy Lim, "Who Should be Subsidised?" *TODAY*, 14 Jan. 2013.

22. dpa news, "Health Insurance to be Mandatory for Foreign Workers in Singapore," *Digital Journal*, 13 Sept. 2007. Available at http://www.digitaljournal.com/article/228017. Ministry of Manpower, "New $15,000 Minimum for Foreign Worker Medical Insurance," 2010. Available at http://mom.gov.sg/newsroom/Pages/HighlightsDetails.aspx?listid=11. L.K. Lee, T.L. Thein et al., "Dengue Knowledge, Attitudes, and Practices among Primary Care Physicians in Singapore," *Ann Acad Med Singapore* 40, 12 (2011): 533–6.

23. Meeting with Dr. Sarah Muttitt, then Chief Information Officer at the Information Systems Division, MOH Holdings, 15 Feb. 2011.
24. See your doctor over a webcam; Lea Wee, "Telemedicine Can Help Save Time and Money without Lowering the Level of Care in Some Medical Situations," *Straits Times*, 23 Feb. 2012.
25. Lea Wee, "Be It a Stroke, an Eye Problem or a Skin Condition, There is a Telemedicine Service to Help You Save Time and Money," *Straits Times*, 23 Feb. 2012.
26. M.K. Lim, "Quest for Quality Care and Patient Safety: The Case of Singapore," *Quality Safety Health Care* 13 (2004): 71–5.
27. Ministry of Health, "Healthcare Quality Improvement and Innovation (HQI2) Fund. Our Healthcare System: Quality & Innovation." Available at http://www.moh.gov.sg/content/moh_web/home/our_healthcare_system/qualityinnovation/HealthcareQualityImprovementandInnovation.html [accessed 1 Apr. 2012].
28. P.N. Chong, N.C. Tan, and T.K. Lim, "Impact of the Singapore National Asthma Program (SNAP) on Preventor-Reliever Prescription Ratio in Polyclinics," *Ann Acad Med Singapore* 37, 2 (2008): 114–7.
29. Health Promotion Board, "Information Paper on Diabetes in Singapore," 14 Nov. 2011. Available at http://www.nrdo.gov.sg/uploadedFiles/NRDO/Publications/%28INP-11-7%29%2020111103%20Diabetes%20Information%20Paper%202011.pdf.
30. Ministry of Health, Singapore, *Health Facts 2007* (Singapore: Ministry of Health, 2008).
31. M.P. Toh, H.S. Leong, and B.K. Lim, "Development of a Diabetes Registry to Improve Quality of Care in the National Healthcare Group in Singapore," *Ann Acad Med Singapore* 38, 6 (2009): 546–6.
32. C.H. Lee, H. Choo et al., "Immigrant Status and Disparities in Health Care Delivery in Patients with Myocardial Infarction," *Int J Cardiol* (2011). doi:10.1016/j.ijcard.2011.11.103.
33. M.K. Lim, "Quest for Quality Care and Patient Safety: The Case of Singapore," *Quality Safety Health Care* 13 (2004): 71–5.
34. M. Niti and T.P. Ng, "Temporal Trends and Ethnic Variations in Amenable Mortality in Singapore 1965–1994: The Impact of Health Care in Transition," *Int J Epidemiol* 30, 5 (2001): 966–73.
35. S.A. Chong, Mythily et al., "Performance Measures for Mental Healthcare in Singapore," *Ann Acad Med Singapore* 37, 9 (2008): 791–6.
36. Speech by former Health Minister Khaw Boon Wan on Mental Health, Special Needs and Traditional Chinese Medicine, 4 Mar. 2011. Available at http://www.thegovmonitor.com/world_news/asia/singapore-highlights-success-of-national-mental-health-blueprint-47276.html.
37. Ministry of Health, "Patient Satisfaction Survey 2010," 2011. Available at http://www.moh.gov.sg/content/moh_web/home/pressRoom/pressRoomItemRelease/2011/Patient_Satisfaction_Survey_2010.html [accessed 19 Mar. 2012].

38. M.K. Lim, "Shifting the Burden of Health Care Finance: A Case Study of Public–Private Partnership in Singapore," *Health Policy* 69, 1 (2004): 83–92.

Chapter 5

1. Pearl Forss, "Public Hospitals Begin Means Testing," *Channel NewsAsia*, 1 Jan. 2009. Available at http://www.channelnewsasia.com/stories/singapore localnews/view/399563/1/.html.
2. Inland Revenue Authority of Singapore website: http://www.iras.gov.sg/irasHome/page04.aspx?id=2110.
3. Hospitals.SG, "Singapore Starts Means Testing in Hospitals," 8 Jan. 2009. Available at http://www.hospitals.sg/story/singapore-starts-means-testing-hospitals.
4. Ministry of Health, "Drug Subsidies. Home: Costs and Financing: Schemes and Subsidies." Available at http://www.moh.gov.sg/content/moh_web/home/costs_and_financing/schemes_subsidies/drug_subsidies.html [accessed 19 Jan. 2012].
5. Y.X. Liew, P. Krishnan et al., "Surveillance of Broad-Spectrum Antibiotic Prescription in Singaporean Hospitals: A 5-Year Longitudinal Study," *PLoS One* 6, 12 (2011): e28751. doi:10.1371/journal.pone.0028751.
6. http://www.moh.gov.sg/content/moh_web/home/pressRoom/pressRoom ItemRelease/2012/revised_healthcaresubsidyratesforpermanentresidents0. html.
7. Singapore Budget 2012 in brief. Available at http://www.singapore budget.gov. sg/budget_2012/download/FY2012_Budget_Highlights.pdf.
8. Budget speech 2012 by Deputy Prime Minister and Minister for Finance M. Tharman Shanmugaratnam. Available at http://www.singaporebudget.gov. sg/budget_2012/budget_speech.html.
9. L. Turner, "'Medical Tourism' and the Global Marketplace in Health Services: U.S. Patients, International Hospitals, and the Search for Affordable Health Care," *Int J Health Serv* 40, 3 (2010): 443–67.
10. Singapore Tourism Board, *Annual Report on Tourism Statistics, 2009* (Singapore: Singapore Tourism Board, 2009), p. 43. Available at https://www.stbtrc.com. sg/images/links/X1Annual_Report_on_Tourism_Statistics_2009.pdf.
11. D. York, "Medical Tourism: The Trend toward Outsourcing Medical Procedures to Foreign Countries," *J Contin Educ Health Prof* 28, 2 (2008): 99–102.
12. http://www.channelnewsasia.com/stories/singaporelocalnews/view/1156836/1/. html.
13. "Booming Medical Tourism Industry," *KPMG Issues Monitor* 7 (2011): 2. Available at http://www.kpmg.com/CH/en/Library/Articles-Publications/Documents/Sectors/pub-20120207-issues-monitor-healthcare-medical-tourism-en.pdf.
14. K.H. Phua, *Privatization and Restructuring of Health Services in Singapore*, Institute of Policy Studies (IPS) Occasional Paper No. 5 (Singapore: IPS, 1991).

15.   http://www.business-in-asia.com/asia/medical_tourism2.html.

16.   L. Lydia and J.R.F. Gan, "Medical Tourism in Singapore: A Structure-Conduct-Performance Analysis," *Journal of Asia-Pacific Business* 12, 2 (2011): 141–70.

17.   Leslie Khoo, *Trends in Foreign Patients Admission in Singapore*, Ministry of Health Singapore Information Paper 2003/01 (Singapore: Ministry of Health, 2003).

18.   Nomura Asia Healthcare Research Team, "Healthcare: Asia Pacific," *Anchor Report*, 9 Dec. 2009, p. 49.

19.   Khoo, *Trends in Foreign Patients Admission in Singapore*. Referenced in Chee Heng Leng, "Medical Tourism and the State in Malaysia and Singapore," *Public Health Ethics* 5 (2012): 38–46.

20.   Josef Woodman, "Patients beyond Borders." Available at http://www1.singapore medicine.com/doc/patients_beyond_borders__singapore_edition_.pdf.

21.   Singapore Hansard, 14 Sept. 2009.

22.   Singapore Hansard, 22 Feb. 2010. Both statements referenced in Chee, "Medical Tourism and the State in Malaysia and Singapore," p. 14.

23.   The Singapore government does not track how its prices for foreign patients in private hospitals compare with other overseas destinations.

24.   http://www.business-in-asia.com/asia/medical_tourism2.html.

Chapter 6

1.   Ministry of Health, "Singapore Healthcare System, 2011." Available at http://www.moh.gov.sg/content/moh_web/home/our_healthcare_system.html [accessed 10 Nov. 2011].

2.   For a list of their services, visit http://www.rafflesmedicalgroup.com/our-services/our-services.aspx.

3.   Adeline Seow L.H.-P., "From Colony to City State: Changes in Health Needs in Singapore from 1950 to 1990," *Journal of Public Health Medicine* 16, 2 (1994): 149–58.

4.   Ministry of Health, "Primary Healthcare Services." Available at http://www.moh.gov.sg/content/moh_web/home/our_healthcare_system/Healthcare_Services/Primary_Care.html [accessed 10 Nov. 2011].

5.   http://www.healthxchange.com.sg/News/Pages/Five-more-poly clinics-to-go-paperless.aspx; http://singaporeseen.stomp.com.sg/stomp/3552/4126/330002]

6.   Polyclinics, Singhealth, "Patient Care." Available at http://polyclinic.singhealth.com.sg/PatientCare/Services/Pages/Home.aspx [accessed 15 Nov. 2011].

7.   National Healthcare Group, "Institutions and Business Divisions." Available at https://corp.nhg.com.sg/Pages/default.aspx [accessed 11 Nov. 2011].

8.   http://www.nuh.com.sg/patients-and-visitors/patients-and-visitors-guide/clinics-and-centres-specialist-outpatient.html.

9.   http://www.moh.gov.sg/content/moh_web/home/pressRoom/pressRoomItem Release/2012/revised_healthcaresubsidyratesforpermanentresidents0.html.

10. L.Y. Wong, B.H. Heng et al., "Using Spatial Accessibility to Identify Polyclinic Service Gaps and Volume of Under-Served Population in Singapore Using Geographic Information System," *Int J Health Plann Manage* 27, 3 (2010): e173–85.

11. http://www.rafflesmedicalgroup.com/clinics/overview.aspx.

12. Ministry of Health, "Primary Care Partnership Scheme." Available at http://www.moh.gov.sg/content/moh_web/home/costs_and_financing/schemes_subisdies/Primary_Care_Partnership_Scheme.html [accessed 16 Nov. 2011].

13. http://www.moh.gov.sg/content/moh_web/home/policies-and-issues/elderly_healthcare.html.

14. Ministry of Health, "Transforming the Primary Care Landscape: Engaging the GP Community and Our Stakeholders in the Journey," 2011. Available at http://www.moh.gov.sg/content/moh_web/home/pressRoom/pressRoom ItemRelease/2011/transforming_theprimarycarelandscapeengagingthe gpcommunityandour.html [accessed 20 Oct. 2011]. Ministry of Health, "Parliamentary QA: Polyclinics," 2011. Available at http://www.moh.gov.sg/content/moh_web/home/pressRoom/Parliamentary_QA/2011/polyclinics.html [accessed 30 Nov. 2011]. Ministry of Health, "Healthcare Services." Available at http://www.moh.gov.sg/content/moh_web/home/our_healthcare_system/Healthcare_Services.html [accessed 16 Nov. 2011].

15. S.P. Ramirez, "A Comprehensive Public Health Approach to Address the Burden of Renal Disease in Singapore," *J Am Soc Nephrol* 14, 7 Supp 2 (2003): S122–6.

16. http://www.nkfs.org/index.php.

17. S.P. Ramirez, T.T. Durai, and S.I. Hsu, "Paradigms of Public–Private Partnerships in End-Stage Renal Disease Care: The National Kidney Foundation Singapore," *Kidney Int Suppl* 83 (2003): S101–7.

18. M.K. Lim, "Transforming Singapore Health Care: Public–Private Partnership," *Ann Acad Med Singapore* 34, 7 (2005): 461–7.

19. Singapore Department of Statistics, *Yearbook of Statistics Singapore, 2011* (Singapore: Singapore Department of Statistics, 2011).

20. Bai Yu, Shi Chaoran, Li Xiaofeng, and Liu Feifei, "Healthcare System in Singapore," *ACTU4625 Topics: Health Insurance*. Available at http://ce.columbia.edu/files/ce/pdf/actu/actu-singapore.pdf.

21. http://www.straitstimes.com/mnt/html/parliament/mar6-GanKimYong-pt1.pdf.

22. Ministry of Health, "Parliamentary QA: Patient Workload in Public Hospitals," 2011. Available at http://www.moh.gov.sg/content/moh_web/home/press Room/Parliamentary_QA/2011/pq27_patient_workloadinpublichospitals-seahkianpeng.html [accessed 23 Nov. 2011].

23. Singapore Department of Statistics, *Yearbook of Statistics Singapore, 2011*.

24. Ministry of Health, "Parliamentary QA: Patient Workload in Public Hospitals."

25. MOH Holdings website: http://www.ahp.mohh.com.sg/our_institutions.html.

26. Ministry of Health, "Singapore Healthcare System, 2011."
27. D. Li, "MOH to Boost Staffing for Long-Term Care," *Business Times*, 19 Aug. 2011.
28. Ministry of Health, "Singapore Healthcare System."
29. Ministry of Health, "Healthcare Regulation." Available at http://www.moh. gov.sg/content/moh_web/home/our_healthcare_system/HealthcareRegulation. html [accessed 30 Aug. 2011].
30. Singapore Medical Council, 2011. Available at http://www.healthprofessionals. gov.sg/content/hprof/smc/en.html [accessed 20 Nov. 2011].
31. MOH Holdings, "About MOH Holdings: Overview." Available at http://www. mohh.com.sg/about_mohh.html [accessed 15 Nov. 2011].
32. D.J. Lim, "The Long Road Ahead for Right-Siting," *Singapore Medical Association News* 39, 4 (2007).
33. Health Promotion Board, "Information Paper on Diabetes in Singapore," 2011, p. 6. Available at http://www.nrdo.gov.sg/uploadedFiles/NRDO/Publications/ %28INP-11-7%29%2020111103%20Diabetes%20Information%20Paper%202 011.pdf.

Chapter 7

1. http://www.singstat.gov.sg/stats/keyind.html.
2. R.M. Nambiar, "Surgical Training—The Challenge of Change," *Ann Acad Med Singapore* 38, 12 (2009): 1034–7.
3. C. Kanchanachitra, M. Lindelow et al., "Human Resources for Health in Southeast Asia: Shortages, Distributional Challenges, and International Trade in Health Services," *Lancet* 377, 9767 (2011): 769–81.
4. http://medicine.nus.edu.sg/corporate/abtus-history.html; http://medicine.nus. edu.sg/corporate/abtus-milestones.html.
5. http://newshub.nus.edu.sg/headlines/0511/qs_04May11.php.
6. National University of Singapore website: http://medicine.nus.edu.sg/ corporate/abtus-transformational_gift.html.
7. http://www.fas.nus.edu.sg/health/.
8. Ibid.
9. For more information, visit http://www.duke-nus.edu.sg/research/signature-research-programs.
10. Interview with Frank Starmer, Associate Dean, Duke-NUS Medical School. See also Frank Starmer, "A Web of Curiosity," *Straits Times*, 25 Aug. 2007.
11. http://www.duke-nus.edu.sg/sites/default/files/research_achievements_ 20111031.pdf.
12. Imperial College London Press Release, 13 Mar. 2012. Available at http:// www3.imperial.ac.uk/newsandeventspggrp/imperialcollege/newssummary/ news_13-3-2012-11-19-17.
13. Ministry of Education Press Release, 2010. Available at http://www.moe.gov. sg/media/press/2010/09/new-medical-school.php.

14. http://www.healthprofessionals.gov.sg/content/hprof/smc/en/leftnav/information_for_registereddoctors/continuing_medical_education/cme_categories.html.

15. http://www.healthprofessionals.gov.sg/content/hprof/smc/en/leftnav/information_for_registereddoctors/continuing_medical_education.html.

16. Nanyang Technological University website: http://www.ntu.edu.sg.

17. http://newshub.nus.edu.sg/headlines/1111/partnering_01Nov11.php.

18. http://www.sph.nus.edu.sg/research/index.html; http://www.sph.nus.edu.sg/news/launch_of_school_of_public_health.html.

19. http://www.spp.nus.edu.sg/Overview_History.aspx.

20. http://www.spp.nus.edu.sg/Research_Centres.aspx.

21. http://newshub.nus.edu.sg/pressrel/1007/100721.php.

22. http://www.gai.nus.edu.sg/research/strategicresearch/NIHA/leadership.html.

23. http://www.gai.nus.edu.sg/aboutus/downloads/GAI%20Brochure.pdf.

24. http://www.gai.nus.edu.sg/aboutus/downloads/GAI%20Brochure.pdf; http://www.gai.nus.edu.sg/aboutus/index.html.

25. http://www.spp.nus.edu.sg/ips/research.aspx.

26. Sree Kumar and Sharon Siddique, "The Singapore Success Story." Available at http://www.eclac.org/publicaciones/xml/1/38981/Singapore_public_private_alliance_innovation_serie_99.pdf.

27. http://www.a-star.edu.sg/AboutASTAR/ASTARJointCouncil/tabid/73/Default.aspx.

28. http://www.a-star.edu.sg/AboutASTAR/Overview/tabid/140/Default.aspx.

29. http://www.a-star.edu.sg/AwardsScholarships/ScholarshipsAttachments/ForGraduatePhDStudies/ASTARGraduateScholarshipOverseas/tabid/202/Default.aspx; http://www.a-star.edu.sg/Portals/0/Awards/forms_brochures/AGS_Brochure.pdf.

30. NIHA Forum: Singapore, Nov. 2010. Khaw Boon Wan, "The Art and Science of Health Care Policy."

31. http://www.pharmaceutical-technology.com/projects/biopolis/.

32. http://www.a-star.edu.sg/tabid/108/default.aspx.

33. Dr. Beh Swan Gin, "Singapore —The Biopolis of Asia," *SMA News* 36, 11 (2004).

34. AsiaOne Business: http://www.asiaone.com/Business/News/SME+Central/Story/A1Story20110127-260718.html; http://www.jtc.gov.sg/Industries/Biomedical/Biopolis/Pages/Biopolis.aspx; http://www.keppeldhcs.com.sg/news_item.aspx?sid=3256.

35. http://www.spring.gov.sg/enterpriseindustry/bhs/pages/industry-background-statistics.aspx.

36. http://www.edb.gov.sg/edb/sg/en_uk/index/industry_sectors/pharmaceuticals__/facts_and_figures.html.

37. http://www.parkwaypantai.com/Library/1/Pages/60/1. Parkway Pantai Limited. pdf.

38. http://epublishbyus.com/ebook/ebook?id=10017047#/12.

39. http://rafflesmedicalgroup.com.sg/ImgCont/626/RMG-AR2011-%20 Commitment-and-Trust.pdf; http://www.rafflesmedicalgroup.com/about-us/ overview.aspx.
40. http://www.swfinstitute.org/swfs/temasek-holdings/.
41. http://www.dancewithshadows.com/business/pharma/pharma-biotech-funds. asp; http://www.prnewswire.com/news-releases/temasek-holdings-to-invest-25-million-in-vical-56566327.html; http://dealcurry.com/20101224-Temasek-Holdings-Buys-3-In-Max-India.htm. Major companies in Temasek's portfolio can be accessed at http://www.temasekreview.com.sg/portfolio/major_ companies.html.
42. Y.J. Zhao, L.C. Tan et al., "Economic Burden of Parkinson's Disease in Singapore," *Eur J Neurol.* 18, 3 (2011): 519–26.
43. http://www.gic.com.sg/global-reach/our-investments.
44. Ministry of Health, *MOH Funds for Healthcare Ideas: In Pursuit of Clinical Excellence* (Singapore: Ministry of Health, 2012).

Chapter 8

1. Lee Hsien Loong , "Preparing for an Aging Population: The Singapore Experience," *The Journal* (Winter 2009). Available at http://www.nus entrepreneurshipcentre.sg/userfiles/files/AARPjournalwinter09_PMLee.pdf.
2. http://www.mcys.gov.sg/successful_ageing/report/CAI_report.pdf.
3. C. Malhotra, A. Chan et al., "Fifteen Dimensions of Health among Community-Dwelling Older Singaporeans," *Curr Gerontol Geriatr Res.* vol. 2011, Article ID 128581, 9 pages (2011). doi:10.1155/2011/128581.
4. J. Phua, A.C. Kee et al., "End-of-Life Care in the General Wards of a Singaporean Hospital: An Asian Perspective," *J Palliat Med.* 14, 12 (2011): 1296–301; Z.J. Ho, L.K. Radha Krishna et al., "Chinese Familial Tradition and Western Influence: A Case Study in Singapore on Decision Making at the End of Life," *J Pain Symptom Manage* 40, 6 (2010): 932–7.
5. N. Venketasubramanian and C.L. Chen, "Burden of Stroke in Singapore," *Int J Stroke* 3, 1 (2008): 51–4.
6. J.P. Thompson and C.M. Riley et al., "Future Living Arrangements of Singaporeans with Age-Related Dementia," *Int Psychogeriatr.* 24, 10 (2012): 1592–9.
7. M. Vimita, "More Eldercare Facilities to be Built over 5 Years," *Channel NewsAsia*, 28 Sept. 2012. Available at http://www.channelnewsasia.com/stories/ singaporelocalnews/view/1228565/1/.html.
8. "Ministerial Committee to Spearhead Successful Ageing for Singapore." Available at http://app.msf.gov.sg/PressRoom/MinisterialCommitteeTo SpearheadSuccessfulAgei.aspx.
9. Speech by Mr Gan Kim Yong, Minister for Health, at the Ministerial Committee on Ageing (MCA) Aged Care Sector Stakeholder's Dialogue on Friday 20 Jan. 2012. Available at http://www.moh.gov.sg/content/ moh_web/home/pressRoom/speeches_d/2012/speech_by_mr_gankimyong ministerforhealthattheministerialcommitte.html.

10. Agency for Integrated Care, "Message from CEO." Available at http://www. aic.sg/page.aspx?id=126.
11. The Agency for Integrated Care website: http://www.aic.sg.
12. http://www.cel.sg/About_CEL__The-LivEnabled-Campaign.aspx.
13. http://www.cel.sg/.
14. http://app.reach.gov.sg/Data/adm05%5CcC6%5Cp5143%5CWorking%20Draf t%20of%20Blueprint-For%20consultation-6%20Oct.pdf.
15. http://www.moh.gov.sg/content/moh_web/home/policies-and-issues/elderly_ healthcare.html.
16. http://www.aic.sg/uploadedFiles/Our_Initiatives/For_Patients_and_ Caregivers/Factsheet%20for%20SPICE_FINAL.pdf; http://www.aic.sg/page. aspx?id=757.
17. Fann Sim, "Health Ministry to Proceed with Eldercare Centre in Woodlands," *Yahoo! News*, 14 Feb. 2012. Available at http://sg.news.yahoo.com/health-ministry-to-proceed-with-eldercare-centre-in-woodlands.html.
18. http://www.tsaofoundation.org/.
19. M. Singh, "Health and Health Policy in Singapore," *ASEAN Economic Bulletin* 16, 3 (1999): 330–43.
20. http://www.mom.gov.sg/employment-practices/employment-rights-conditions/ cpf/Pages/cpf-life.aspx.
21. http://mycpf.cpf.gov.sg/Members/Gen-Info/CPF_LIFE/CPF_LIFE.htm; http://mycpf.cpf.gov.sg/CPF/my-cpf/reach-55/SubPage.htm; http://mycpf. cpf.gov.sg/NR/rdonlyres/09EA0C05-C8E9-4705-9D91-E8BD1D12CF1E/0/ LIFEBrochure.pdf?NRMODE=Unpublished&wbc_purpose=Basic&WBCM ODE=PresentationUnpubliished.
22. Poon Chian Hui, "More Affordable Long-Term Care for Patients," *Straits Times*, 18 Feb. 2012.
23. Gerald C.H. Koh, "A Review of Geriatric Education in Singapore," *Annals Academy of Medicine* 36, 8 (2007): 687–90.
24. http://www.sna.org.sg/site/gerontological/gerontological-2.html.
25. D. Li, "MOH to Boost Staffing for Long-Term Care," *Business Times*, 19 Aug. 2011.
26. Singapore Department of Statistics, "Statistics: Households and Housing (Themes)," 2011. Available at http://www.singstat.gov.sg/stats/themes/people/ household.html [accessed 20 Nov.2011].
27. http://www.hpb.gov.sg/HOPPortal/health-article/10176?_afrLoop= 22019147807756239&_afrWindowMode=0&_afrWindowId=5w9vtpsmi_ 1#%40%3F_afrWindowId%3D5w9vtpsmi_1%26_afrLoop%3D2201914780 756239%26_afrWindowMode%3D0%26_adf.ctrl-state%3D5w9vtpsmi_17.

Bibliography

Government Publications

Committee on Ageing Issues. *Report on the Ageing Population*. Singapore: MCYS, 2006. Available at http://www.mcys.gov.sg/successful_ageing/report/CAI_report.pdf.

Health Promotion Board. "Information Paper on Diabetes in Singapore," 14 Nov. 2011. Available at http://www.nrdo.gov.sg/uploadedFiles/NRDO/Publications/%28INP-11-7%29%2020111103%20Diabetes%20Information%20Paper%202011.pdf.

Khoo, Leslie. *Trends in Foreign Patients Admission in Singapore*. Ministry of Health Singapore Information Paper 2003/01. Singapore: Ministry of Health, 2003.

Ministry of Health. *Affordable Health Care—A White Paper*. Singapore: Singapore National Printers for the Ministry of Health, 1993, p. 70.

———, Epidemiology and Disease Control Department. *National Health Survey 2004*. Singapore: Ministry of Health, 2005.

———. *Health Facts 2007*. Singapore: Ministry of Health, 2008.

———. *Our Quality Journey: Singapore's Healthcare Milestones*. Singapore: Ministry of Health, 2010.

Ministry of Social and Family Development. "Ministerial Committee to Spearhead Successful Ageing for Singapore," 4 Mar. 2007. Available at http://app.msf.gov.sg/PressRoom/MinisterialCommitteeToSpearheadSuccessfulAgei.aspx.

National Population and Talent Division. *A Sustainable Population for a Dynamic Singapore: Population White Paper, January 2013*. Singapore: National Population and Talent Division, 2013. Available at http://202.157.171.46/whitepaper/downloads/population-white-paper.pdf.

Singapore Cancer Registry. *Cancer Survival in Singapore 1968–2007*. Singapore: Health Promotion Board, 2011.

Singapore Department of Statistics. *Yearbook of Statistics Singapore, 2011*. Singapore: Singapore Department of Statistics, 2011.

Singapore Tourism Board. *Annual Report on Tourism Statistics*, 2009. Singapore: Singapore Tourism Board, 2009.

Books and Articles

Barr, M.D. "Medical Savings Accounts in Singapore: A Critical Inquiry." *J Health Polit Policy Law* 26, 4 (2001): 709–26.

Beh Swan Gin. "Singapore —The Biopolis of Asia." *SMA News* 36, 11 (2004).

"Booming Medical Tourism Industry." *KPMG Issues Monitor* 7 (2011): 2. Available at http://www.kpmg.com/CH/en/Library/Articles-Publications/Documents/Sectors/pub-20120207-issues-monitor-healthcare-medical-tourism-en.pdf.

Boyd, Jennifer B., Mary H. McGrath, and John Maa. "Emerging Trends in the Outsourcing of Medical and Surgical Care." *JAMA Surgery* 146, 1 (2011): 107–12.

Chee Heng Leng. "Medical Tourism and the State in Malaysia and Singapore." *Public Health Ethics* 5 (2012): 38–46.

Chee, Y.C. "Do No Harm: Do Thyself No Harm, 2005 SMA Lecture." *Singapore Med J* 46, 12 (2005): 667.

Chong, S.A., Mythily et al. "Performance Measures for Mental Healthcare in Singapore." *Ann Acad Med Singapore* 37, 9 (2008): 791–6.

Chong, P.N., N.C. Tan, and T.K. Lim. "Impact of the Singapore National Asthma Program (SNAP) on Preventor-Reliever Prescription Ratio in Polyclinics." *Ann Acad Med Singapore* 37, 2 (2008): 114–7.

dpa news. "Health Insurance to be Mandatory for Foreign Workers in Singapore." *Digital Journal*, 13 Sept. 2007. Available at http://www.digitaljournal.com/article/228017.

Dong, W. "Can Health Care Financing Policy be Emulated? The Singaporean Medical Savings Accounts Model and Its Shanghai Replica." *J Public Health* 28, 3 (2006): 209–14.

Emmanuel, S.C., S.L. Lam et al. "A Countrywide Approach to the Control of Non-Communicable Diseases—The Singapore Experience." *Ann Acad Med* 31, 4 (2002): 474–8.

Fordham, Margaret. "The Law of Negligence." Available at http://www.singaporelaw.sg/content/Negligence.html

Gauld, R., N. Ikegami et al. "Advanced Asia's Health Systems in Comparison." *Health Policy* 79, 2–3 (2006): 325–36.

Hin, C.C. "Planning for the Future—The National Health Plan." *Singapore Med J* 28, 3 (1987): 210–3.

Ho, Z.J., L.K. Radha Krishna et al. "Chinese Familial Tradition and Western Influence: A Case Study in Singapore on Decision Making at the End of Life." *J Pain Symptom Manage* 40, 6 (2010): 932–7.

Hospitals.SG. "Singapore Starts Means Testing in Hospitals." Hospitals.SG., 8 Jan. 2009. Available at http://www.hospitals.sg/story/singapore-starts-means-testing-hospitals.

Kanchanachitra, C., M. Lindelow et al. "Human Resources for Health in Southeast Asia: Shortages, Distributional Challenges, and International Trade in Health Services." *Lancet* 377, 9767 (2011): 769–81.

Karvounis, Niko. "Health Care in Singapore." In *Taking Note: A Century Foundation Group Blog*. Available at http://takingnote.tcf.org/2008/07/health-care-in.html.

Knight, B. "No-Fault Compensation and Performance Review." *Ann Acad Med Singapore* 22, 1 (1993): 61–4.

Koh, Gerald C.H. "A Review of Geriatric Education in Singapore." *Annals Academy of Medicine* 36, 8 (2007): 687–90.

Lee, C.H., H. Choo et al. "Immigrant Status and Disparities in Health Care Delivery in Patients with Myocardial Infarction." *Int J Cardiol* (2011). doi:10.1016/j.ijcard.2011.11.103.

Lee Hsien Loong . "Preparing for an Aging Population: The Singapore Experience." *The Journal* (Winter 2009). Available at http://www.nusentrepreneurshipcentre.sg/userfiles/files/AARPjournalwinter09_PMLee.pdf.

Lee Kuan Yew. *From Third World to First: The Singapore Story 1965–2000*. New York: HarperCollins Publishers, 2000.

Lee, L.K., T.L. Thein et al. "Dengue Knowledge, Attitudes, and Practices among Primary Care Physicians in Singapore." *Ann Acad Med Singapore* 40, 12 (2011): 533–6.

Liew, F., L.W. Ang et al. "Evaluation on the Effectiveness of the National Childhood Immunisation Programme in Singapore, 1982–2007." *Ann Acad Med Singapore* 39, 7 (2010): 532–10.

Liew, Y.X., P. Krishnan et al. "Surveillance of Broad-Spectrum Antibiotic Prescription in Singaporean Hospitals: A 5-Year Longitudinal Study." *PLoS One* 6, 12 (2011): e28751. doi:10.1371/journal.pone.0028751.

Lim, D.J. "The Long Road Ahead for Right-Siting." *Singapore Medical Association News* 39, 4 (2007).

Lim, J.F. and V.D. Joshi. "Public Perceptions of Healthcare in Singapore." *Ann Acad Med Singapore* 37, 2 (2008): 91–5.

Lim, Linette. "P&G Invests $250m in Innovation Centre." *The Business Times*, 27 Jan. 2011. Available at http://www.asiaone.com/Business/News/SME+Central/Story/A1Story20110127-260718.html.

Lim M.K. "Health Care Systems in Transition II. Singapore, Part I. An Overview of Health Care Systems in Singapore." *Journal of Public Health Medicine* 20, 1 (1998): 16–22. Available at http://jpubhealth.oxfordjournals.org/content/20/1/16.full.pdf.

———. "Quest for Quality Care and Patient Safety: The Case of Singapore." *Quality Safety Health Care* 13 (2004): 71–5.

———. "Shifting the Burden of Health Care Finance: A Case Study of Public–Private Partnership in Singapore." *Health Policy* 69, 1 (2004): 83–92.

———. "Transforming Singapore Health Care: Public–Private Partnership." *Ann Acad Med Singapore* 34, 7 (2005): 461–7.

———. "Transforming Singapore Health Care: Public–Private Partnership." *Ann Acad Med Singapore* 34, 7 (2005): 461–7.

Lim, Y.P. "Sharing Singapore's Experience in Dietetic Practice and School Nutrition Programmes." *Asia Pac J Clin Nutr* 17, Supp 1 (2008): 361–4.

Lydia, L. and J.R.F. Gan. "Medical Tourism in Singapore: A Structure-Conduct-Performance Analysis." *Journal of Asia-Pacific Business* 12, 2 (2011): 141–70.

Malhotra, C., A. Chan et al. "Fifteen Dimensions of Health among Community-Dwelling Older Singaporeans." *Curr Gerontol Geriatr Res* vol. 2011, Article ID 128581, 9 pages (2011). doi:10.1155/2011/128581.

Nambiar, R.M. "Surgical Training—The Challenge of Change." *Ann Acad Med Singapore* 38, 12 (2009): 1034–7.

National Coalition on Health Care. "Health Care Spending as Percentage of GDP Reaches All-Time High." 12 Sept. 2011. Available at http://nchc.org/node/1171.

Nomura Asia Healthcare Research Team. "Healthcare: Asia Pacific." *Anchor Report*, 9 Dec. 2009, p. 49.

Niti, M. and T.P. Ng. "Temporal Trends and Ethnic Variations in Amenable Mortality in Singapore 1965–1994: The Impact of Health Care in Transition." *Int J Epidemiol* 30, 5 (2001): 966–73.

Organisation for Economic Co-operation and Development (OECD). *Health at a Glance: Asia/Pacific 2010.* Paris: OECD, 2010.

OECD. *Health at a Glance 2009: OECD Indicators.* Paris: OECD 2009, p. 200.

Parkway Holdings 2010 Report Card. Available at http://epublishbyus.com/ebook/ebook?id=10017047#/12.

Parkway Pantai Limited Fact Sheet. Available at http://www.parkwaypantai.com/Library/1/Pages/60/1. Parkway Pantai Limited.pdf.

"Partnering One of the World's Leading Institutions in Global and Pulbic Health." *Newshub—NUS' News Portal*, 1 Nov. 2011. Available at http://newshub.nus.edu.sg/headlines/1111/partnering_01Nov11.php.

Phua, J., A.C. Kee et al. "End-of-Life Care in the General Wards of a Singaporean Hospital: An Asian Perspective." *J Palliat Med* 14, 12 (2011): 1296–301.

Phua Kai Hong. *Privatization and Restructuring of Health Services in Singapore.* Institute of Policy Studies (IPS) Occasional Paper No. 5. Singapore: IPS, 1991.

———. "Attacking Hospital Performance on Two Fronts: Network Corporatization and Financing Reforms in Singapore." In *Innovations in the Delivery of Health Services: The Corporatization of Public Hospitals,* ed. A.S. Preker and A. Harding. Washington, DC: World Bank, 2003, pp. 7–9. Available at http://books.google.com/books?id=iFIVuwFa7GEC&pg=PA468&lpg=PA468&dq=revenue+caps+at+Singapore+public+hospitals&source=bl&ots=v5l7Vmi4oF&sig=ZTg_4Z8spwAxkG1xaafMZYpA_KI&hl=en&sa=X&ei=IizOT8jwNIX76gGjqayxDA&ved=0CHEQ6AEwBg#v=onepage&q=revenue%20caps%20&f=false.

———. *Social Health Insurance: Selected Case Studies from Asia and the Pacific.* WHO South East Asia Region, New Delhi and Western Pacific Region, Manila, 2005.

Poon, W.O. "Malpractice and Negligence in the Medical Professions." *Singapore Med J* 24, 3 (1983).

Ramesh, M. "Autonomy and Control in Public Hospital Reforms in Singapore." *The Americal Review of Public Administration* 38, 1 (2008): 18.

Ramirez, S.P. "A Comprehensive Public Health Approach to Address the Burden of Renal Disease in Singapore." *J Am Soc Nephrol* 14, 7 Supp 2 (2003): S122–6.

Ramirez, S.P., T.T. Durai, and S.I. Hsu. "Paradigms of Public–Private Partnerships in End-Stage Renal Disease Care: The National Kidney Foundation Singapore." *Kidney Int Suppl* 83 (2003): S101–7.

Sankaranarayanan, R., R. Swaminathan et al. "Cancer Survival in Africa, Asia, and Central America: A Population-Based Study." *Lancet Oncology* 11, 2 (2010): 165–73.

Seow, Adeline L.H.-P. "From Colony to City State: Changes in Health Needs in Singapore from 1950 to 1990." *Journal of Public Health Medicine* 16, 2 (1994): 149–58.

Schreyögg, Jonas and Lim Meng Kin. "Health-Care Reforms in Singapore—Twenty Years of Medical Savings Accounts." *CESifo DICE Report*, Ifo Institute for Economic Research at the University of Munich 2, 3 (Oct. 2004): 55–60.

Singh, M. "Health and Health Policy in Singapore." *ASEAN Economic Bulletin* 16, 3 (1999): 330–43.

Sree Kumar and Sharon Siddique. "The Singapore Success Story." Available at http://www.eclac.org/publicaciones/xml/1/38981/Singapore_public_private_alliance_innovation_serie_99.pdf.

Thompson, J.P. and C.M. Riley et al. "Future Living Arrangements of Singaporeans with Age-Related Dementia." *Int Psychogeriatr* 24, 10 (2012): 1592–9.

Toh, C.M., S.K. Chew, and C.C. Tan. "Prevention and Control of Non-Communicable Diseases in Singapore: A Review of National Health Promotion Programmes." *Singapore Med J* 43, 7 (2002) 333–9.

Toh, M.P., H.S. Leong, and B.K. Lim. "Development of a Diabetes Registry to Improve Quality of Care in the National Healthcare Group in Singapore." *Ann Acad Med Singapore* 38, 6 (2009): 546–6.

Turner, L. "'Medical Tourism' and the Global Marketplace in Health Services: U.S. Patients, International Hospitals, and the Search for Affordable Health Care." *Int J Health Serv* 40, 3 (2010): 443–67.

United States Agency for International Development. "Medical Malpractice Law 'Best Practices' for Jordan." 21 Aug. 2007.

Venketasubramanian, N. and C.L. Chen. "Burden of Stroke in Singapore." *Int J Stroke* 3, 1 (2008): 51–4.

Wong, L.Y., B.H. Heng et al. "Using Spatial Accessibility to Identify Polyclinic Service Gaps and Volume of Under-Served Population in Singapore Using Geographic Information System." *Int J Health Plann Manage* 27, 3 (2010): e173–85.

Woodman, Josef. "Patients beyond Borders." Available at http://www1.singaporemedicine.com/doc/patients_beyond_borders__singapore_edition_.pdf.

World Health Organization. *The World Health Report 2000 Health Systems: Improving Performance*. Geneva: WHO, 2000.

York, D. "Medical Tourism: The Trend toward Outsourcing Medical Procedures to Foreign Countries." *J Contin Educ Health Prof* 28, 2 (2008): 99–102.

Bai Yu, Shi Chaoran, Li Xiaofeng, and Liu Feifei. "Healthcare System in Singapore." *ACTU4625 Topics: Health Insurance*. Available at http://ce.columbia.edu/files/ce/pdf/actu/actu-singapore.pdf.

Zhao, Y.J., L.C. Tan et al. "Economic Burden of Parkinson's Disease in Singapore." *Eur J Neurol* 18, 3 (2011): 519–26.

News Articles

Boon, G.T. "Provident Fund Gets a Big Welcome." *The Singapore Free Press*, 1 Dec. 1953, p. 12. Available at http://newspapers.nl.sg/Digitised/Article/freepress 19531201.2.55.aspx.

Forss, Pearl. "Public Hospitals Begin Means Testing." *Channel NewsAsia*, 1 Jan. 2009. Available at http://www.channelnewsasia.com/stories/singaporelocalnews/view/399563/1/.html.

"Impressed that Polyclinic Waiting Time Cut Down by More Than Half." Available at http://singaporeseen.stomp.com.sg/stomp/3552/4126/330002.

Khalik, Salma. "Doctors from Abroad form Growing Pool in Singapore." *Asiaone*, 19 Aug. 2009. Available at http://www.asiaone.com/Health/News/Story/A1Story20090818-161867.html.

_____. "Medisave Can be Used in 12 M'sian Hospitals." *Straits Times*, 15 Feb. 2010. Available at http://www.asiaone.com/Health/News/Story/A1Story20100216-198974.html.

_____. " Cervical Cancer Jabs Covered by Medisave." *Straits Times*, 5 Oct. 2010.

_____. "Easier to Bring in Foreign-Trained Docs." *Straits Times*, 26 Mar. 2011. Available at http://www.healthxchange.com.sg/News/Pages/Easier-to-bring-in-foreign-trained-doctors.aspx.

_____. "Health Subsidies Extended to 710,000." *Straits Times*, 16 Aug. 2011, p. 2.

Khan, Irfan. "Temasek Holdings Buys 3% In Max India." *DealCurry*, 24 Dec. 2010. Available at http://dealcurry.com/20101224-Temasek-Holdings-Buys-3-In-Max-India.htm.

Li, D. "MOH to Boost Staffing for Long-Term Care." *Business Times*, 19 Aug. 2011.

Lim, Jeremy. "Who Should be Subsidised?" *TODAY*, 14 Jan. 2013.

Mohandas, Vimita. "Singapore Medical Tourism Booming." *Channel NewsAsia*, 2 Oct. 2011.

_____. "Budget: Medifund, MediShield to be Enhanced to Relieve High Medical Costs." *Channel NewsAsia*, 17 Feb. 2012. Available at http://www.channelnews asia.com/stories/singaporelocalnews/view/1183628/1/.html.

Ng, Julia. "Lasik Prices Expected to Fall Further when Pte Sector Publishes Bill Sizes." *Channel NewsAsia*, 8 Feb. 2008. Available at http://www.channelnews asia.com/stories/singaporelocalnews/view/327682/1/.html.

"NUS Medicine Ranks First in Asia in QS World University Rankings®." *Newshub—NUS' News Portal*, 4 May 2011. Available at http://newshub.nus.edu.sg/headlines/0511/qs_04May11.php.

"NUS Spearheads New Initiative to Advance Public Health and Healthcare Delivery in Asia." *Newshub—NUS' News Portal*, 21 July 2010. Available at http://newshub.nus.edu.sg/pressrel/1007/100721.php/.

Poon Chian Hui. "Five More Polyclinics to Go Paperless." *Straits Times*, 5 Mar. 2011. Available at http://www.healthxchange.com.sg/News/Pages/Five-more-polyclinics-to-go-paperless.aspx.

_____. "More Affordable Long-Term Care for Patients," *Straits Times*, 18 Feb. 2012.

Ro, Sam. "Revealed: The Cost of Health Insurance around the World." *Business Insider*, 26 Apr. 2012. Available at http://www.businessinsider.com/cost-of-health-insurance-around-the-world-2012-4#ixzz1zZizuLFo.

Runckel, Charles. "Where to Go for Medical Tourism?" Available at http://www.business-in-asia.com/asia/medical_tourism2.html.

Saad, Imelda. "Singapore Unveils S$2b Package to Boost Fertility Rate." *Channel NewsAsia*, 21 Jan. 2013. Available at http://www.channelnewsasia.com/stories/singaporelocalnews/view/1249234/1/.html.

Sim, Fann. "Health Ministry to Proceed with Eldercare Centre in Woodlands." *Yahoo! News*, 14 Feb. 2012. Available at http://sg.news.yahoo.com/health-ministry-to-proceed-with-eldercare-centre-in-woodlands.html.

Starmer, Frank. "A Web of Curiosity." *Straits Times*, 25 Aug. 2007.

Tan Weizhen. "ElderShield Scheme Review Will Not Be Rushed." *TODAY*, 30 Apr. 2012.

"Temasek Holdings to Invest $25 Million in Vical." *PR Newswire*, 19 Oct. 2006. Available at http://www.prnewswire.com/news-releases/temasek-holdings-to-invest-25-million-in-vical-56566327.html.

Vimita, M. "More Eldercare Facilities to be Built over 5 Years." *Channel NewsAsia*, 28 Sept. 2012. Available at http://www.channelnewsasia.com/stories/singapore localnews/view/1228565/1/.html.

Wee, Lea. "Telemedicine Can Help Save Time and Money without Lowering the Level of Care in Some Medical Situations." *Straits Times*, 23 Feb. 2012.

_____. "Be It a Stroke, an Eye Problem or a Skin Condition, There is a Telemedicine Service to Help You Save Time and Money." *Straits Times*, 23 Feb. 2012.

Websites

A*STAR

http://www.a-star.edu.sg/tabid/108/default.aspx

http://www.a-star.edu.sg/AboutASTAR/Overview/tabid/140/Default.aspx

http://www.a-star.edu.sg/AboutASTAR/ASTARJointCouncil/tabid/73/Default.aspx

http://www.a-star.edu.sg/AwardsScholarships/ScholarshipsAttachments/For GraduatePhDStudies/ASTARGraduateScholarshipOverseas/tabid/202/Default.aspx; http://www.a-star.edu.sg/Portals/0/Awards/forms_brochures/AGS_Brochure.pdf

Agency for Integrated Care

http://www.aic.sg

http://www.aic.sg/page.aspx?id=126.

http://www.aic.sg/uploadedFiles/Our_Initiatives/For_Patients_and_Caregivers/Factsheet%20for%20SPICE_FINAL.pdf; http://www.aic.sg/page.aspx?id=757

Central Provident Fund

http://ask-us.cpf.gov.sg/explorefaq.asp?category=23069

http://ask-us.cpf.gov.sg/Home/Hybrid/themes/CPF/Uploads/Healthcare/General
   Information on MSH.pdf

http://ask-us.cpf.gov.sg/exploreMQA.asp?projectid=1734594&category=23071&str
   page=0&strPrint=#4185193

http://askus.cpf.gov.sg/Home/Hybrid/themes/CPF/Uploads/Healthcare/General%
   20Information%20on%20MSH.pdf

http://mycpf.cpf.gov.sg/CPF/my-cpf/have-child/HC2.htm

http://mycpf.cpf.gov.sg/CPF/News/News-Release/N_11May2012.htm

http://mycpf.cpf.gov.sg/NR/rdonlyres/78E52772-ED48-4477-9167-28A31
   DE2566B/0/CPFTrends_Medishield.pdf

http://mycpf.cpf.gov.sg/NR/rdonlyres/B9577B11-693D-4E34-A83D-123E1
   F7731D4/0/MedisaveScheme_Trends_March2011.pdf

http://mycpf.cpf.gov.sg/Members/Gen-info/WIS/WIS_Scheme.htm

http://mycpf.cpf.gov.sg/Members/Gen-Info/CPF_LIFE/CPF_LIFE.htm; http://
   mycpf.cpf.gov.sg/CPF/my-cpf/reach-55/SubPage.htm; http://mycpf.cpf.
   gov.sg/NR/rdonlyres/09EA0C05-C8E9-4705-9D91-E8BD1D12CF1E/0/
   LIFEBrochure.pdf?NRMODE=Unpublished&wbc_purpose=Basic&WBC
   MODE=PresentationUnpubliished

Centre for Enabled Living

http://www.cel.sg/

http://www.cel.sg/About_CEL__The-LivEnabled-Campaign.aspx

Health Promotion Board

http://www.hpb.gov.sg/programmes/article.aspx?id=3324

http://www.hpb.gov.sg/HOPPortal/health-article/10176?_afrLoop=220
   1914780756239&_afrWindowMode=0&_afrWindowId=5w9vtpsmi_
   1#%40%3F_afrWindowId%3D5w9vtpsmi_1%26_afrLoop%3D220
   1914780756239%26_afrWindowMode%3D0%26_adf.ctrl-state%
   3D5w9vtpsmi_17

Housing and Development Board

http://www.hdb.gov.sg/fi10/fi10320p.nsf/w/AboutUsHDBHistory?OpenDocument

International Institute for Strategic Studies

http://www.iiss.org/about-us/

http://www.iiss.org/about-us/offices/iiss-asia-singapore/

Medical Protection Society

http://www.medicalprotection.org/singapore/aboutmps/discretion

http://www.medicalprotection.org/Default.aspx?DN=31cbb51f-e7d4-4feb-9769-ea30cb040ab5

Ministry of Health

http://www.moh.gov.sg/mohcorp/pressreleases.aspx?id=25992

http://www.moh.gov.sg/content/moh_web/home/pressRoom/pressRoomItem Release/2001/hepatitis_B_immunisation_programme.html

http://www.moh.gov.sg/content/moh_web/home/pressRoom/pressRoomItem Release/2009/use_of_medisave_for_pneumococcal_vaccination.html

http://www.moh.gov.sg/content/moh_web/home/pressRoom/pressRoomItem Release/2011/Patient_Satisfaction_Survey_2010.html

http://www.moh.gov.sg/content/moh_web/home/pressRoom/highlights/2011/10_top_common_myths_of_singapore_health_care.html

http://www.moh.gov.sg/content/moh_web/home/pressRoom/pressRoomItem Release/2011/extending_medisaveforscreeningmammogramsand colonoscopies. html

http://www.moh.gov.sg/content/moh_web/home/pressRoom/pressRoomItem Release/2011/transforming_theprimarycarelandscapeengagingthegpcommunity andour.html

http://www.moh.gov.sg/content/moh_web/home/pressRoom/Parliamentary_ QA/2011/polyclinics.html

http://www.moh.gov.sg/content/moh_web/home/pressRoom/Parliamentary_ QA/2011/pq27_patient_workloadinpublichospitals-seahkianpeng.html

http://www.moh.gov.sg/content/moh_web/home/pressRoom/press RoomItem Release/2012/revised_healthcaresubsidyratesforpermanentresidents0. html

http://www.moh.gov.sg/content/moh_web/home/pressRoom/pressRoomItem Release/2012/revised_healthcaresubsidyratesforpermanentresidents0.html

http://www.moh.gov.sg/content/moh_web/home/pressRoom/speeches_d/2012/ speech_by_mr_gankimyongministerforhealthattheministerialcommitte.html

http://www.moh.gov.sg/content/moh_web/home/costs_and_financing/schemes_ subsidies/drug_subsidies.html

https://http://www.moh.gov.sg/content/moh_web/home/costs_and_financing/ schemes_subsidies/ElderShield.html

https://www.moh.gov.sg/content/moh_web/home/costs_and_financing/schemes_ subsidies/ElderShield/ElderShield_Supplements.html

http://www.moh.gov.sg/content/moh_web/home/costs_and_financing/schemes_ subsidies/Marriage_and_Parenthood_Schemes.html

http://www.moh.gov.sg/content/moh_web/home/costs_and_financing/schemes_ subsidies/medisave.html

http://www.moh.gov.sg/content/moh_web/home/costs_and_financing/schemes_ subsidies/Medifund.html

http://www.moh.gov.sg/content/moh_web/home/costs_and_financing/schemes_
    subsidies/Medifund/Eligibility.html
http://www.moh.gov.sg/content/moh_web/home/costs_and_financing/schemes_
    subsidies/MediShield/How_MediShield_Works.html
http://www.moh.gov.sg/content/moh_web/home/costs_and_financing/schemes_
    subisdies/Primary_Care_Partnership_Scheme.html
http://www.moh.gov.sg/content/moh_web/home/our_healthcare_system.html
http://www.moh.gov.sg/content/moh_web/home/our_healthcare_system/Healthcare_
    Services/Primary_Care.html
http://www.moh.gov.sg/content/moh_web/home/our_healthcare_system/
    qualityinnovation/HealthcareQualityImprovementandInnovation.html
http://www.moh.gov.sg/content/moh_web/home/our_healthcare_system/Healthcare
    Regulation.html
http://www.moh.gov.sg/content/moh_web/home/our_healthcare_system/Healthcare_
    Services.html
http://www.moh.gov.sg/content/moh_web/home/policies-and-issues/elderly_
    healthcare.html
http://www.moh.gov.sg/content/moh_web/home/statistics/Health_Facts_Singapore/
    Disease_Burden.html
http://www.pqms.moh.gov.sg/apps/fcd_faqmain.aspx?qst=2fN7e274RAp%2BbUzL
    dEL%2FmJu3ZDKARR3p5Nl92FNtJiewnENBNFEIiRHmMoeVHrwwzG
    A%2BwFOVoSHTBVPEq9DECk2raoDSEH38mKUHHqhk8DNKUlN0L
    EZB7u5R8QnS8ViteA1ZHO8%2FJ69cMiJ3pMFKfSbDdcjb9lI1j7OsjaVpX
    P7wy%2F5C36hQHIXBtwt%2BNFxi9CoSAkmphWY%3D

Ministry of Manpower

http://mom.gov.sg/newsroom/Pages/HighlightsDetails.aspx?listid=11
http://mom.gov.sg/employment-practices/employment-rights-conditions/cpf/Pages/
    cpf-life.aspx

MOH Holdings

http://www.ahp.mohh.com.sg/our_institutions.html
http://www.mohh.com.sg/about_mohh.html

Nanyang Technological University

http://www.ntu.edu.sg

National Healthcare Group

https://corp.nhg.com.sg/Pages/default.aspx
http://www.nhgp.com.sg/ourservices.aspx?id=5000000013
http://www.nhg.com.sg/nhg_01_pressRelease2003_5july.asp?pr=2003

National University of Singapore

http://www.duke-nus.edu.sg/research/signature-research-programs
http://www.duke-nus.edu.sg/sites/default/files/research_achievements_20111031.
    pdf
http://www.fas.nus.edu.sg/health/
http://www.gai.nus.edu.sg/aboutus/downloads/GAI%20Brochure.pdf
http://www.gai.nus.edu.sg/aboutus/index.html.
http://medicine.nus.edu.sg/corporate/abtus-history.html
http://medicine.nus.edu.sg/corporate/abtus-milestones.html
http://medicine.nus.edu.sg/corporate/abtus-transformational_gift.html
http://www.sph.nus.edu.sg/news/launch_of_school_of_public_health.html.
http://www.sph.nus.edu.sg/research/index.html
http://www.gai.nus.edu.sg/research/strategicresearch/NIHA/leadership.html
http://www.spp.nus.edu.sg/ips/research.aspx.
http://www.spp.nus.edu.sg/Overview_History.aspx
http://www.spp.nus.edu.sg/Research_Centres.aspx

Raffles Medical Group

http://www.rafflesmedicalgroup.com/clinics/overview.aspx
http://www.rafflesmedicalgroup.com/our-services/our-services.aspx
http://rafflesmedicalgroup.com.sg/ImgCont/626/RMG-AR2011-%20Commitment-
    and-Trust.pdf

Singapore Budget

http://www.singaporebudget.gov.sg/budget_2012/budget_speech.html
http://www.singaporebudget.gov.sg/budget_2012/download/FY2012_Budget_
    Highlights.pdf

Singapore Department of Statistics

http://www.singstat.gov.sg/stats/keyind.html
http://www.singstat.gov.sg/stats/keyind.html#birth
http://www.singstat.gov.sg/stats/themes/economy/hist/gdp1.html
http://www.singstat.gov.sg/stats/themes/people/household.html

Singapore Medical Council

http://www.healthprofessionals.gov.sg/content/hprof/smc/en.html
http://www.healthprofessionals.gov.sg/content/hprof/smc/en/leftnav/information_
    for_registereddoctors/continuing_medical_education/cme_categories.html
http://www.healthprofessionals.gov.sg/content/hprof/smc/en/leftnav/information_
    for_registereddoctors/continuing_medical_education.html

Others

https://www.babybonus.gov.sg/bbss/html/index.html

http://www.edb.gov.sg/edb/sg/en_uk/index/industry_sectors/pharmaceuticals__/
facts_and_figures.html

http://www.geraldtan.com/premed/Doctor_salaries.html

http://www.gic.com.sg/global-reach/our-investments

http://www.growandshare.gov.sg/Overview.htm

http://gstvoucher.gov.sg/

http://www3.imperial.ac.uk/newsandeventspggrp/imperialcollege/newssummary/
news_13-3-2012-11-19-17

http://www.income.com.sg/insurance/i-Medicare/index.asp

http://www.iras.gov.sg/irasHome/page04.aspx?id=2110.

http://www.mof.gov.sg/budget_2011/key_initiatives/families.html

http://www.indexmundi.com/singapore/total_fertility_rate.html

http://www.jtc.gov.sg/Industries/Biomedical/Biopolis/Pages/Biopolis.aspx

http://www.keppeldhcs.com.sg/news_item.aspx?sid=3256

http://www.moe.gov.sg/media/press/2010/09/new-medical-school.php

http://www.nkfs.org/index.php.

http://www.nuh.com.sg/patients-and-visitors/patients-and-visitors-guide/clinics-
and-centres-specialist-outpatient.html

http://www.patient-help.com/

http://www.pharmaceutical-technology.com/projects/biopolis/

http://polyclinic.singhealth.com.sg/PatientCare/Services/Pages/Home.aspx

http://pss.org.sg

http://www.sna.org.sg/site/gerontological/gerontological-2.html

http://www.spring.gov.sg/enterpriseindustry/bhs/pages/industry-background-
statistics.aspx

http://www.singaporemedicalguide.com/hospital-ward-classes/

http://www.singaporemedicine.com/abt_us/abt_us1.asp

http://www.swfinstitute.org/swfs/temasek-holdings

http://www.temasekreview.com.sg/portfolio/major_companies.html

http://www.tsaofoundation.org/

Index